Fasting a Spiritual Discipline with Physical Benefits
Cleansing the Holy Spirit's Temple

Fasting a Spiritual Discipline with Physical Benefits

Fasting a Spiritual Discipline with Physical Benefits
Cleansing the Holy Spirit's Temple

Terri Flynn

Fasting a Spiritual Discipline with Physical Benefits

Copyright © 2015 by Terri Flynn.

Scriptures quotations taken from www.biblegateway.com

Scripture quotations marked ESV are from The Holy Bible, English Standard Version® copyright © 2001 by Crossway, a publishing ministry of Good News Publishers. Used by permission.

Scripture quotations marked GW are taken from GOD'S WORD®, © 1995 God's Word to the Nations. Baker Publishing Group. Used by permission.

Scripture quotations marked KJV are taken from the King James Version of the Bible, Public domain.

Scripture quotations marked NASB are taken from the NEW AMERICAN STANDARD BIBLE ®, Copyright ©

The Master Cleanser published in 1976 Stanley Burroughs published.

An application to register this book for cataloging has been submitted to the Library of Congress.

ISBN- 13: 978-1515327264 Soft cover
ISBN- 10: 1515327264 E-Book

https://www.createspace.com/ 5653724

Printed in the United States of America

Terri Flynn

Dedication

I dedicate this book to the many individuals who are struggling to lose weight and to those who have been on the weight loss roller coaster. Have faith that you can trust in God's help and live within normal and healthy weight limits. Through fasting and healthy eating, you can restore your temple to look and feel as God created it to be.

Contents

Preface

My Struggle

I have spent most of my life struggling with eating properly, stuck in a constant cycle of indulging, then gaining weight, starving myself and then losing weight. I have repeated this cycle over, and over again for forty plus years. Long before I was a teenager I have been worried about being fat, which resulted in some really unhealthy dieting habits; very often not eating at all. My story began early on when I was around nine years old. My friend Patty and I both had older brother and they would always tease us and call us fat. It was then when we started fasting, but not for spiritual reason. In realty we were on starvation diets. As I look back at photos of us there was not a bit of fat on either of us. From that point on how I saw myself and how much I weight has always been an ongoing struggle for me. Even when I was at my thinnest I would still look in the mirror and think that I was fat.

For far too many years I would put on and take off anywhere for ten-fifteen pounds it was a continuous up and down weight battle. However, the last eight years has been the toughest battle for me. When I met my husband Sean I wanted to give myself a break and I promised myself I would not step on the scale again because it had such a powerful hold on me. Unfortunately my promise worked against me and I ended up gaining thirty-seven pounds in our first seven years of marriage and I had been trying to take it off unsuccessfully. I knew it was time to give up foods that triggered my unhealthy eating habits. That is how I came up with this weight loss cleanse.

Terri Flynn

Chapter 1

Making a Change

For too many years I have been so obsessed with my weight. I was tired of the endless dieting cycle, I wanted to take back my body and start eating right, especially now that I am getting older I need to be more cautious about what and when I eat. I knew it was time to start focusing less on what I weighted and start making wiser food choices. 1 Corinthians 10:31 tells us, "*So, whether you eat or drink, or whatever you do, do everything to the glory of God.*" I have made the resolution that we're made to consume food, food was never meant to control us.

I made a decision this year to really make a change. I have made the choice to eat mostly green foods, fruits, vegetables and fish. In Genesis 1:29, God said, "*I am giving you all the grain bearing plants and all the fruit trees. These trees make fruit with seeds in it. This grain and fruit will be your food.*" I knew it was time to give up foods that triggered my unhealthy eating habits, so I gave up deserts first. I quickly noticed that I had more energy and just felt better.

Since my body was reacting poorly to certain foods. I decided to give up sugar, and not just the white sugar, but anything that turned in to sugar in my body or that was processed. I also stopped eating dairy, red meats, and anything with glutens in them. Since I removed these foods from my diet I have noticed a physical and emotional improvement in my body. I am no longer bloated or

1

inflamed. I can think clearer and it has helped me to lose weight and keep it off.

A lot of people that choose to go gluten free start using gluten free products that have become more available in the grocery store. I believe that it is better to stay away from those gluten free boxed products since they are all processed. They will quickly put the weight back on you. I talk more about a gluten free diet in chapter eight.

It is better to choose foods like raw fruits and vegetables they are very low in calories, so you can eat more food and feel more satisfied. A nice fresh salad with a vinaigrette dressing and lemon water would be a good choice. You would be satisfied and still have a lot of calories left for the rest of the day. Make it an aim to eat as much healthy food as you can and still stay within your calorie goal.

We don't get healthy accidental. It takes a deliberate effort, it's a choice, and it requires a lifestyle change. But it begins with a declaration. For long time success, a lifestyle change is a must if you are overweight. You won't change until you choose to change. It takes more than desire to get healthy it takes a decision. Ephesians 4:22 tells us, "*You were told that your foolish desires will destroy you and that you must give up your old way of life with all its bad habits.*" If changing your eating and exercise habits is something you cannot stick with then your weight loss will be temporary.

Everyone wants to be healthy, but very few people choose to be healthy. Long time success requires making wise choices. Deuteronomy 2:3 tells us, *"You have traveled around these mountains long enough. Turn north."* If you have been stuck in a vicious cycle of defeat; it's time to follow God's directions into the Promised Land of freedom from food addiction. Remember everyone is different so find something that works for you and make the commitment to stick with it. Then once you lose the weight to maintain your desired weight you must stick to new eating habits.

When I was a teenager, my girlfriend and I were always dieting. We had a saying you may have heard it "nothing taste as good as skinny feels." I still feel that way today.

When I am in my healthy weight range I feel fabulous. So I remind myself regularly that living in victory will be tastier than any food I could be eating right now. I also realize that my food choices matter to God, and I am accountable for how I treat my body that is another reason I choose to make healthy eating habits. Romans 14:12 tells us, "Each of us will give an account of ourselves to God."

The simple facts about weight gain or loss is if we consume more calories than we burn up in exercise, we will gain weight and if we burn up more calories in exercise than we consume in food then we will reduce our weight. A lifestyle change requires a new way of thinking. If we want to change how we act, we must begin by changing the way we think and talk. The way we think and talk controls the way we feel, and the way we feel controls our actions. That is why a lifestyle change requires God's help. It is only with the help of Jesus that we can change. The Holy Spirit can and will help us break free from bad

3

eating habits, compulsion eating, and food addictions when we ask Him for His guidance and help.

Our bodies are a temple; a gift from God. We will be blessed when we care for our bodies. By eating healthy we are getting the energy and nutrition our bodies need to function to its full potential. My girlfriend would also say, "A moment on our lips is a lifetime on our hips." Even at a young age we realized that an act that took a minute could remain with us forever. The weigh is always easier to put on than it is to get off. We could also apply that saying to prayer. A moment of prayer on our lips can change our lives, our behavior, and our hearts for a long time. A simple prayer can change us, can lead us on the path to health, and healing. We need to ask God to give us knowledge and strength to keep our bodies strong and healthy. Then we will have no need to ask Him to heal a sick and diseased body that we created ourselves by not taking care of the Holy Spirit's temple.

Our hunger for food is a physical reminder of how much we really need God. Just like our bodies need nourishment and water to maintain life, we also need spiritual food to pursue holiness and see God clearly. It is time that we become hungry for holiness. 1 Corinthians 6:20 tells us, *"God paid a very high price to make you His. So honor God with your body."* When we change the way we eat we are honoring God with our bodies. This will take determination but it is possible with God's help. It is time we realize that we are either building strong healthy bodies from healthy and nutritious foods to honor God or we are building diseased bodies from unhealthy foods which dishonors the Holy Spirit's temple.

4

Since our bodies are the Holy Spirit's temple, our goal should be to find a way to take care for our body and treat them with respect. Three things need to happen to achieve this. Exercising regularly, stop overeating, and learn to fast from the food that are not healthy for us. When we remove unhealthy foods from our diet we are taking caring of the Holy Spirit's temple. As a result, we will decrease our weight. Then when we have achieved an ideal weight we should fast those unhealthy foods continuously, in order to maintain that ideal weight.

Put Food in it Proper Place

It is time that food received an appropriate place in our life. Food is a gift from God for nourishment and energy, food should not be used as our source of comfort. When we run to the cabinet to eat away our problems, or treat ourselves to a daily ice cream, cookie or a mac attack, food turns into something more than it was ever meant to be. Psalm 16:11 tells us, "*You make the path of life known to me. Complete joy is in your presence."* When Jesus is the focus of our joy and comfort we are able to put food in its appropriate place in our lives.

Our habits are important if we want to accomplish victory. Because our habits governor our lives. Exchanging poor eating habits for healthy eating habits is essential for a permanent lifestyle change. Since our habits have been established over a long period of time. Changing them will take some hard work. Remember weight loss is by no means simple or quick. So often we want to improve our health and we start out with eagerness and anticipation but a few days or weeks later those feelings disappear and so does our resolution.

Keep in mind we live in a microwave world and weight loss is like a crook-pot or a slow-cooker. That is why ongoing victory requires us to develop new healthy eating and exercise practices. Positive habits that replace our unhealthy behaviors. You might be overweight, an overeater, or have some type of eating disorder, whatever the case no one got that way overnight. Those habits were established over a long period of time. To change a habit we need to cultivate a whole new pattern of thinking. It is only through the strength of Jesus that I found victory. Psalm 28:7 tells us, *"The Lord is my strength and shield. I trusted Him with all my heart He helped me, so I am happy. I sing songs of praise to Him."*

Terri Flynn

Chapter 2

Losing Weight with God

In Christ

We often think our habits identify who we are. However, they are not our identity but they may have been rooted from our childhood. I know that my adult habits were established in my childhood. For some people unhealthy habits may have developed because of unmet emotional needs or to soothe negative feelings started at a young age. It is important to remember that habits are things we do not who we are and habits can be replaced. Instead of complaining about how unfortunate I was to have a slow metabolism, or that I suffered from an eating disorder, or whining that I failed at yet another weight-loss attempt. I changed my outlook. Now I see myself as a child of God; a forgiven, accepted, victorious, and loved women of God. Proverbs 14:1 tells us, *"The wise woman builds her house, but the foolish tears it down with her own hands."* To develop healthy habits you need to begin to build yourself up in what God says about you, and accept who you are in Christ. Start seeing yourself as God sees you.

It is essential to know and live by our true identity in Christ. If you want to eat healthy but find yourself in battle of defeat, try changing your thoughts with God's empowering Scriptures. Scriptures can become fresh nourishment to shape your thoughts that will start you on your journey to permanent success. Keep in mind God has made us for much more than being caught in unhealthy eating habits that leaves us feeling conquered and enslaved. You were created to be free, confident, and victorious. As you read these Scriptures accept your true identity as a child of God.

Scripture on Your True Identity in Christ

We are children of God - John 1:12 (ASV) *"But as many as received Him, to them gave he the right to become children of God, even to them that believe on His name."*

We are chosen by God - 1 Peter 2:9 (NCV) *"But you are a chosen people, royal priests, a holy nation, a people for God's own possession. You were chosen to tell about the wonderful acts of God, who called you out of darkness into His wonderful light."*

We are loved by God - Romans 8:37 (CEB) *"But in all these things we win a sweeping victory through the one who loved us."*

We are forgiven of sins - Ephesians 1:7 (NET Bible) *"In Him we have redemption through His blood, the forgiveness of our trespasses, according to the riches of His grace."*

We are strengthened by Christ - Philippians 4:13 (ERV) *"Christ is the one who gives me the strength I need to do whatever I must do."*

We have the Holy Spirit's help - John 14:16 (ESV) *"And I will ask the Father, and He will give you another Helper, to be with you forever."*

We have peace with God - Romans 5:1 (NIV) *"Therefore, since we have been justified through faith, we have peace with God through our Lord Jesus Christ."*

There is no condemnation in us - Romans 8:1 (GNT) *"There is no condemnation now for those who live in union with Christ Jesus."*

We are a new creation in Christ - 2 Corinthians 5:17 (MEV) *"Therefore, if any man is in Christ, he is a new creature. Old things have passed away. Look, all things have become new."*

We are chosen - Ephesians 1:11 (NIRV) *"We were also chosen to belong to Him. God decided to choose us long ago in keeping with His plan. He works out everything to fit His plan and purpose."*

We have access to God - Ephesians 3:12 (RSV) *"In whom we have boldness and confidence of access through our faith in Him."*

We are light to the world - Ephesians 5:8 (HCSB) *"For you were once darkness, but now you are light in the Lord. Walk as children of light."*

We are rooted in Christ - Colossians 2:7 (CEV) *"Plant your roots in Christ and let Him be the foundation for your life. Be strong in your faith, just as you were taught. And be grateful."*

We are new in Christ - Colossians 3:3 (ERV) *"Your old self has died, and your new life is kept with Christ in God."*

The Holy Spirit's Temple

Our bodies are the temple of the Holy Spirit. Each are uniquely designed by our Creator. God intends for us to care for and treat these temples properly. 1 Corinthians 6:19-20 tells us that, *"You should know that your body is a temple for the Holy Spirit that you received from God and that lives in you. You don't own yourselves. [20] God paid a very high price to make you his. So honor God with your body."* Even though one day we will answer to God for the way in which we treat our bodies, He still gives us the freedom to decide how we will take care of them. That being said, our bodies need to consume nutritious food for energy every day. We also need to give our bodies the appropriate amount of sleep and exercise.

Once I got the revelation that God gave me, this temple and I need to keep it healthy. That part of His love for me is His desire for me to be healthy. I knew if I wanted to transform both my physical and spiritual health, I would need to come up with a healthy eating program. I was going to have to go to Scripture and develop my own program based on God's Words. I realized if I wanted to eat healthy and not once again find myself in battle of defeat, it was time to replace food with Jesus. This time I am not losing weight for me but to honor the body God has given me.

12

Strength from God

Once I understood how much I needed Jesus to help me conquer this long life struggle. I recognized that not only does God care about this struggle in my life, but knowing that His grace is sufficient for me has changed the way I look at my struggle with my weight. He loves me and is compassionate about my circumstances. 2 Corinthians 12:9 tells us *that, "My grace is sufficient for you: for my strength is made perfect in weakness."* I also realized that I could not change my habits or my life while depending on my own strength.

Maintaining a healthy weight is a daily process. I wake up every morning with a choice to honor God with my body that day or not. I know that I was made for more and that each choice I make determines my victory or defeat spiritually, mentally, and physically. It has to become a lifestyle change that is meant to be carried on every day. For it to work it is going to take a complete dependence on Jesus. I realized that learning to hunger for Jesus instead of food, has abundant benefits and the way I care for my body is a part of my witness daily. Philippians 4:1 tells us, *"Christ is the one who gives me the strength I need to do whatever I must do."* I am confident that I can defeat this struggle through the strength that Jesus gives me. With the Holy Spirit guiding my every choice I will continue my journey to where there will be a healthier leaner me.

For a long time I knew that I had an eating issue. I have tried many different diet and read countless books on the subject of dieting. I have fasted with my church on a twenty one day fast since 2000. Many years I extended the fast to forty days. Even though by the end of the fast I was lighter, as soon as I started eating again, I put the weight back on and many years a few pounds more. I had an eye-opening revelation that my struggle wasn't about food and my weakness wasn't about a lack of will power. It was about the way that I saw myself. Jesus is doing an amazing work in my head and heart and I'm experiencing freedom in my thought life. As I have learned to depend on Jesus when I feel weak, He continues to answer my prayers when I ask for His help with strength and discipline.

I ask Jesus daily to be my portion of strength, patience and wisdom. He has shown me that every day I need to lay down the strongholds that bound me for so long and I need to take hold of His promises. God's Word has opened my eyes and more importantly my heart to the truths I desperately needed to hear to become free of my food struggles. This entire journey has led me to be stronger and close in the Lord. I know that success can be a reality when Jesus is a part of it for that reason, He must be the in center of this life long journey, for victory to be mine. That is why I has chosen to make these changes and to love the body God gave me and care for it well. Jesus is our portion; He really is all we need. Lamentations 3:24 tells us that, *"My portion is the Lord, I have said to myself, so I will put my hope in Him."*

Honor God with Your Body

The Bible doesn't directly mention weight loss, however, there is a lot in God's Word about the importance of taking care of our bodies and our health. In Deuteronomy 14, God told the Israelites in depth about what they were and were not to eat.   Most of these commands God gave were to keep them from eating foods that would harm their health. The Lord wants His children to take excellent care of their bodies since they are the home of the Holy Spirit.   A strong, healthy body helps us stay in shape so we can better serve God each day and this brings glory and honor to Him.   Some days will be easier than others but keep in mind that your body is not your own and you honor God with the way you choose to treat it.   Pray about making healthy food choices and Jesus will revealed Himself to you as your refuge, your healer, and your sustainer. Most importantly you will begin to feel closer to Jesus and sense Him right beside you helping you make healthier choices. You are not alone and with the Lord's help you will win this battle.

I challenge you to seek Jesus more than food. It is time to make the commitment to get out of the destructive weight loss and gain cycle. I hope that this book will give you the tools to change your perspective and hunger for Jesus instead of food.   We are woman of God and He wants us to be free of unhealthy food choices and the destruction that the weight loss and gain cycle does to our bodies and emotions. I hope to encourage you to win your personal food and exercise wars.

It is time to declare that I am not losing weight for me, but for Jesus and He has satisfied my hungers. As long as you continue to stay focused on His Word, your faith will grow and you will be victorious this time around. As a result of focusing on God's promises you will gain more confidence in yourself, with Godly self-esteem and most importantly self-discipline. Jesus will change you in ways you never even knew were possible.

Repenting

We must also take in to consideration that to constantly obsess about food, exercise, diet, and weight loss means we've allowed our bodies to become the center of our lives. When we become obsessed with weight loss and our body image our bodies have become an idol in our lives. If we place anything as a major focus in life and it isn't Jesus, it is sin. The Lord wants us to keep our focus on Him and not fall into obsessing about weight gain and weight loss. I have had to repent from my obsession of how much I weigh. It was only by sincerely humble myself before the Lord, repenting, praying, meditating on His Word and consistently seeking God's face that my stronghold was broken and He brought me through this obsession.

It is so important not to let our appetites control us, but we are to have control over our appetites. Proverbs 28:7 tells us, *"Whoever follows God's teachings is a wise son. Whoever associates with gluttons disgraces his father."* Gluttony seems to be one of those sin that many Christians like to overlook. Many believers would not ever consider harming their body through putting unhealthy things like alcohol, cigarette, or drugs in their body but have no guilt about stuffing themselves with food. But overeating or indulging in too much foods is gluttony, which the Bible says is a sin. If you have harmed your body through gluttony, confess it as sin to God and repent.

Self-control

Controlling our diet is one of the hardest undertakings we encounter in life. Throughout Scripture many have failed to control their appetite with tragic results such as Adam and Esau. One of the fruits of the Spirit is self-control, Galatians 5:22-23 tells us, *"But the fruit that the Spirit produces in a person's life is love, joy, peace, patience, kindness, goodness, faithfulness, 23 gentleness, and self-control."* The ability to say "no" to anything in excess is self-control. God wants us to control our appetites, rather than allowing it to control us. We need to begin to limit our portions to the right amounts of food and remove unhealthy and processed foods from our daily diets. God has blessed us with a large variety of foods that are nutritious, and delicious. We should honor God by enjoying these foods and by eating them in appropriate amounts.

Taking Action

It is only by the strength of God that we can do anything successfully. Speaking God's Word and prayer is an important part of that strength. However, we can recite all the Scripture we can find and pray to God for help concerning weight loss, but if we do not take action and make a change we will not see any lasting results.

Every time there is a miracles mentioned in the Bible, action was required. When God divided the Red Sea, He instructed Moses to raise his staff. When Jesus anointed the eyes of the blind man with the clay, He instructed the man to go and wash in the pool of Siloam. Elisha sent a messenger to tell the King of Israel to go and wash seven times in the Jordan. They all had to take action. So ask God daily for wisdom on the appropriate actions to take to lose weight.

We need to put our faith into action every day. Hebrews 6:12 tells us, *"We don't want you to be lazy. We want you to be like those who, because of their faith and patience, will get what God has promised."* According to Scripture, we will inherit the promises of God when we put faith and patience in action. Losing weight will take a lot of patience and a lot of effort. Now that you are asking God for wisdom to help you lose weight and get healthy consider what the Word of God says about these things. Use what His Word says about health as affirmations. Then continue to thank God daily for helping you put them in to action.

God's Word instructs us to do what we know is right. James 4:17 tells us, *"If you fail to do what you know is right, you are sinning."* We all should know some good things to do that will help our body stay healthy. Most of us know that junk food is unhealthy it is food that is high in calorie and nutrient poor. These poor nutrition foods are related to heart problems, high blood pressure, and a host of other health related diseases.

Also sugar is the single worst ingredient in our diets. It can have harmful effects on metabolism and contribute to all sorts of diseases. Refined sugar, sucrose, and high fructose corn syrup which are in many processed foods contain a whole bunch of calories with no essential nutrients. There are no proteins, essential fats, vitamins or minerals in sugar just pure energy and empty calories.

A Cleanse Helps Our Bodies Detox

Excess weight is often a result of consuming foods that do not work for our individual body, resulting in poor digestion and toxic overload. Often our bodies will not begin to shed extra weight until it has found balance through the cleansing process. During a cleanse we start to re-balance the acidity and alkaline in our bodies and repair the damage done by years of poor eating habits. When we lose weight without cleansing the toxins out first; the weight-loss typically doesn't last very long. It is important to take into account that everybody has a different level of toxicity so weight-loss will occurs at a different speed for everyone.

During a detox cleanse many people may feel more emotional than usual. This is because cleansing is not just about the body since we are also spirit and soul. I will talk more about the difference between our spirit, soul, & body in chapter three. When we detox we also release emotional toxins. So spend time in pray reflecting on your emotions and ask Jesus to help you release the unhealthy eating habits once and for all.

Daily Fourteen Hours Fast

A daily fourteen hours fast will also help you get the most out of your cleanse and is also a good daily practice when you are not on a cleanse. A daily fourteen hours fast starts after your evening meal, you will leave at least a fourteen hour window before having your morning meal. If you have your evening meal at 6 pm, you should have your morning meal no sooner than at 8 am. Keep in mind when we fill up our stomach late at night, and eat early again the next day, we are not giving our bodies the opportunity to digest all of our food properly.

Terri Flynn

Chapter 3

The Holy Spirit's Help

Spirit, Soul, & Body

Our spirit is what gets born again; when we put our faith in Jesus our spirit is recreated. God takes out our old spirit and He puts in a brand new one. Our spirit is filled with the Holy Spirit that is why our bodies are the His temple. 1 Thessalonians 5:23 tells us, *"We pray that God himself, the God of peace, will make you pure belonging only to Him. We pray that your whole self; spirit, soul, and body will be kept safe and be blameless when our Lord Jesus Christ comes."* We are fabulously fashioned by God. He made us in a way that our spirit, soul, and body are all connected and work together perfectly according to His design.

Fasting is a spiritual discipline with physical benefits. Fasting should always merge with a spiritual purpose. During a fast we want to put our spirit in control of our soul and body. The goal is for our bodies to establish new healthy eating and lifestyle habits that are controlled by our spirit.

Our soul is significantly affected during a fast and often it is not very happy with our sudden change in diet. Especially if our eating habits were unhealthy before the fast. 3 John 1:2 tells us, *"Beloved, I pray that you may prosper in all things and be in health, just as your soul prospers."* This is an indication of the importance of attending to matters of the soul as it relates to being healthy.   The soul is where our character emotions, intellect, and will are.   It is where we experience our

23

feelings. In the Bible, the soul is referred to as our flesh. Fasting is not always an easy discipline to practice. Going without food can be a struggle especially for those not familiar to it. Triumphing over this struggle with our flesh is one of the most powerful rewards of a fast.

During a fast our bodies are transformed as our diet is changed. During the first few days you may experience headaches, moodiness, and fatigue. Because you are going through a detox period. Your bodies may experience withdrawal from a number of unhealthy things. Such as, sugar, chemicals, caffeine, fats, and food additives. After a few days these symptoms will subside. Also during a fast many people experience healing and most people lose weight. Of course how much we lose is determined on what foods we are eating. If we eat a lot of nuts, bean, and potatoes on a fast we will probably not lose much weight and might even gain some.

The basic cause of disease is the habits of improper diet, not enough exercise, negative mental attitudes, and lack of spiritual understanding. Which produces toxic conditions and breakdown of our bodies. By developing proper habits physically 'body', mentally 'soul', and spiritually 'spirit' you will experience health and healing in all three of these areas of your life.

While fasting you may experience breakthroughs in your spirit, soul, and body; below are some of the benefits often experience.

Spirit

A closer relationship with God
Sensitive to hear God's voice
Helps us to rely on God's strength
Spiritual breakthrough
A new desire for God
A deeper praise

Soul

Nourishes positive emotions
Frees our mind of negative thoughts
Brings peace
Overcome negative habits
Breaks addictions to unhealthy foods

Body

Detoxification our body organs
Jump starts healthy weight loss
Improves skin
Improves memory and attention span
Reduces stress
Promotes restful sleep
Aids in digestion
Reduces inflammation
Enhances immune system

Endless the Diet Cycle

If you are tired of the endless diet cycle, it is time to replace food that contain artificial ingredients or comes from a cardboard box, a can, a bag, or a fast food restaurant with the things God placed on this earth to feed His children. For example fruits, vegetables, nuts, seeds, health whole grains, fish, and lots of water. A good way to end the diet cycle is to start that change is with a fast.

Fasting

Fasting does not always mean to do without food entirely. Fasting is doing without foods that we do not really need or foods that has a control over our life. In addition, fasting does not mean that we should deprive yourselves of nutrition. As you fast you are applying self-control by turn down unhealthy food you once enjoyed or thought that you needed.

Jesus has made us to hunger for Him. If we depend on food to satisfy us, we will only feel temporary fulfillment because we will only become empty again. When will begin to hunger for a closer relationship with Jesus we discover how to become completely fulfilled. By drawing closer to Jesus through fasting, prayer, and speaking His Word over our health we will begin to enjoy spiritual healing that will satisfy our soul and our hunger allowing us to break free of all the harmful habits that have been damaging our health.

While you are fasting, ask Jesus to satisfy your hunger and give you the desire to be healthy. Matthew 5:6 tells us, *"Blessed are those who hunger and thirst for righteousness, for they shall be satisfied."* Use your hunger as a motivation to pray instead of picking up a chip or a cookie.   Ask Jesus to encourage you to find fulfillment in nutritious food choices.

Fasting when combined with prayer achieves a powerful means to draw closer to Jesus. When we make prayer a habit before we put unhealthy food in our mouth the Holy Spirit will give us the desire and self-discipline to escape the urge. Remember that the Bible teaches us that we are a spirit, we have a soul and we live in a body, which is the Holy Spirit's temple. When we fast it has an effect on all three parts of us.

Through fasting and prayer we achieves a powerful means to draw closer to Jesus and we learn how to satisfy our desires for Him instead of food. He will encourage us when we want to eat unhealthy food choices. It is also an awesome time to teach ourselves to focus on and seek after Jesus for His wisdom and help with our weight struggle.

During a fast is a great time to feed on Biblical truth. By reading the Bible daily and committing to memory Scriptures that can help you see yourselves as God sees you. After all we are God's masterpiece. Ephesians 2:10 tells us, *"For we are God's masterpiece. He has created us anew in Christ Jesus, so we can do the good things He planned for us long ago."* It is so important to know and accept our true identity in Christ and acknowledge who we are and whose we are by accepting our identity.

Do not rush into your fast make a promise to yourself and to God ahead of time. It is also important to prepare yourself before you begin a fast. Start by eating smaller meals and stay away from fatty and sugary foods. A few days before the fast eat more fruit and vegetables. Write down what you plan on eating and omitting. If you have health concerns that need consideration check with your physician before going on any fast.

When you do a fast you will begin to feel healthier physically, spiritually, and mentally. Any type of fasting should remind us that we are nourished by every word that proceeds out of the mouth of God. The purpose of fasting is to abstain from food for the purpose of transforming our life to know and hear Jesus more. Romans 12:2 tells us, *"Don't be conformed to the patterns of this world, but be transformed by the renewing of your minds so that you can figure out what God's will is what is good and pleasing and mature."* Fasting is a great way to transform our spirit, soul and, body. As we endure through the early mental and physical uneasiness, we will undergo an uplifting in our soul and decline in the hunger.

In addition, fasting also produces many health benefits as well as spiritual. Fasting leads to weight loss, which is good for most people because most people are overweight. Fasting can also promote detoxification, improve our immune system, decreases inflammation, even out blood sugar, lowers blood pressure, and gives our digestive system a chance to relax. When you fast unto the Lord, you can look forward to a supernatural resource of energy.

Terri Flynn

Chapter 4

Fasting to Lose Weight

A change of diet can be the first step to a healthier lifestyle. Fasting to lose weight might be the push that is needed to get your diet started. Fasting triggers detoxification; a healing process which allows the body to naturally cleanse itself. An unhealthy diet that's high in fat, sugars, and processed foods lets harmful bacteria accumulate which slows down the digestive systems and interfere with elimination, allowing harmful toxins to build up in the colon and arteries. As a result, some of the poor health that can develop related to toxicity are cancer, cardiovascular disease, arthritis, allergies, obesity, skin problems, headaches, fatigue, pains, coughs, inflammation, and gastrointestinal issues.

Fasting with a well-balanced whole food vegetarian diet can help cleanse the body and can eventually eliminate many of the harmful effects of toxic foods. When we eliminate high-fat foods, sugars, meat, and processed foods from our diet, a considerable amount of our body's energy is freed from the intense work of digesting these foods. Detoxification and cleansing the body of harmful toxins is a huge benefit of a whole foods vegetarian diet. When we begin eating a more healthy vegetarian diet, we start to get more dietary fiber into our systems and our digestive systems start to work as it should. In addition, the dietary fiber found in whole foods, such as fruits, vegetables, nuts, and legume helps fill you up and keeps you feeling full longer so you eat less.

Liquid Fast

A liquid fast is a wonderful way to jump start a cleanse. A liquid fast can consists of water but this is not usually recommended for more than a few days. Another way to do a liquid fast is consuming foods that are in liquid state as a sources of nutrition while excluding any solid foods. Food consumed during a liquid fast may include items like smoothie's, juices, pureed soups, tea, and plenty of water. Liquid fasts are easier on your digestion system than solid foods. Also if you are going to consume a liquid fast to lose weight, you will need to make sure you are still getting a good balance of nutrients throughout the day and consuming a proper amount of calories for your weight loss goal.

It is possible to get the nutrition you need while consuming a liquid fast and you can continue to stay on this fast for long periods of time. The nutrients in whole food juices will provide energy and support your body while speeding up the detoxification process and releasing waste from your systems. Keep in mind you will need to make sure you get enough fiber during your liquid fast otherwise you can wind up suffering from constipation.

Once you are ready to transition back to solid foods you will need to be careful not to gain all of the weight back. A good way to do that is to transition over to a whole food fast for a while. A whole food fast is a diet that is low in calories so you can continue to manage your weight loss during this transition period. The Daniel fast is a wonderful way to continue your weight loss program. In addition you can choose to include the whole food liquid diet, which is essentially a Daniel fast in liquid form for 1 or 2 meals as you slowing start adding more healthy solid whole foods as part of your fast. Transitioning in to the Daniel fast will help you learn healthy eating habits that will make it easier to keep your weight down.

The Daniel Fast

Daniel was a prophet in the Old Testament. The Daniel fast is a partial fast of plant-based nutrition. The first time we hear about the Daniel fast in the Bible was a ten day fast mentioned in the first chapter of Daniel. Daniel did not want to eat the king's rich food and wine because according to Jewish tradition it would make him unclean. Daniel talked to the guard who had been put in charge over him and his friends. Daniel 1:12 tells us, *"He said, Please give us this test for ten days. Don't give us anything but vegetables to eat and water to drink. 13 Then after ten days, compare us with the other young men who eat the king's food. See for yourself who looks healthier, and then decide how you want to treat us, your servants." 14So the guard agreed to test Daniel, Hananiah, Mishael, and Azariah for ten days. 15 After ten days, Daniel and his friends looked healthier than all the young men who ate the king's food."*

The second time we hear about the Daniel fast was a twenty one day fast mentioned in the tenth chapter of Daniel. Daniel had a vision, the message was true and one of great conflict, and he understood the message and had understanding of the vision. Daniel 10:2 tells us, *"In those days I, Daniel, was mourning three full weeks. 3 I ate no tasty food, no meat or wine entered my mouth, nor did I anoint myself at all until three whole weeks were fulfilled."*

The primary reason that God created plant life was to provide a source of food for man and beast. The Daniel fast consists of fruits, vegetables, nuts, grains, and legumes. Although eating meat became permitted after the great flood, plants based foods are still the most beneficial to us.

Getting Started

If you are ready to make the decision to take good care of the body God has given you. Then let's get started with four steps.

Prayer - Pray for the wisdom and strength to make healthy food choices and eat appropriate portions on the fast and as a new life style.

Remember - Remember that your body is a gift from God and it is your responsibility to take good care of it.

Confess - Confession and repentance for miss treating the Holy Spirit's temple.

Stop - Stop drinking coffee and caffeine drinks; slowly cut down. Over the course of a week right before you start the detox program gradually cutting back. For example if you drink four cups of coffee per day, the first day still drink that amount, then on the second day cut back to two cups, on the third day only drink one cup, on the fourth day only drink a half of a cup, and on the fifth day don't have any. This will minimize caffeine withdrawal headaches.

I am thrilled you want to be healthier and I hope you will join me on my journey of permanent weight loss. Weight loss and healing can come from a few simple dietary changes, your body will have a chance to heal, detox and restore; allowing you to notice how good you can really feel.

Keep in mind regardless of what you eat your overall intake of calorie determines how much weight you will lose. For example when I started my weight loss plan I was 149.5, I was sitting most of the day at my computer so I wasn't very active. For me to lose weight without working out I would only be able to consume about 1000 calories per day. That may not sound like a lot of calories however, since I was eating a healthy diet of fruits and vegetable it was quite lot of food and it is completely satisfied. Keep in mind that one pound of body fat equals 3500 calories, and those calories add of quickly when you are eating high fat, sugary, and processed foods.

One way keep track of your calories is by using online programs that are completely free and easy to use they will help you achieve your weight loss goals. I have a list of helpful website in the back of this book.

Chapter 5

Cleansing the Holy Spirits Temple Program

The cleansing program that I have created has three parts and it is a forty day fast. This program is unique because it offers the benefits of fasting, but without totally going without food and nourishment. The first part is an easy detox cleanse and the second and third parts are partial fasts that are fairly easy to follow, which makes it perfect for anyone who has never tried fasting before.

The first part of the detox cleanse program begins with a liquid cleanse of spicy lemon-limeade for the first ten days. The second part consist of a liquid fast on whole food with fresh fruit and vegetable juice, smoothies, pureed soups, and herbal tea for nine days. The third part is the Daniel fast with eating fruits, vegetables, root vegetables, legumes, nuts, seeds for twenty one day. You can also continue with whole food juice, smoothies, soups, and herbal tea, and of course plenty of water during part three.

The spicy lemon-limeade cleanse rids our body of toxins that have built up over the years due to poor eating habits. It is one way of breaking the unhealthy eating cycle. Stanley Burroughs created the lemonade fast also known as the Master Cleanse program in 1940 to cure stomach ulcer. Later in the year 1976, Stanley launched a book about it, stating that this cleansing program not only cures stomach ulcers, but also cleanses the colon, reduces body weight, and also treats other disorders. According to Burroughs, toxins are caused by consuming meat, dairy, drugs, antibiotics, fungus-causing foods, pesticides and all the other junk that we put into our bodies. I agree with him.

My Experience

I began my forty day fast on a detox cleansing program with the spicy lemon-limeade cleanse for ten days. On the cleanse most people will see a large chunk of weight fall off during the ten days. However, that's just starts the ball rolling; when you go off the spicy lemon-limeade you'll find you no longer desire unhealthy foods. Even though you will lose weight during the ten day cleanse, that isn't the goal. The goal is to purge your bodies of toxins that are weighing you down and start fresh. Toxins have been accumulated in our body from the foods that we eat such as meat, processed foods, pesticides, dairy, and fast food. Cleansing will make you want to change your eating habits, and desire more health food like vegetables, fruits, and water.

I saw fast result the first ten days on the cleanse it transform me in to a lighter, younger looking, and more energetic version of myself. In the first ten days of my cleanse I lose ten lbs. I woke up every morning well rested and feeling better than the night before. The spicy lemon-limeade flushed out waste and restore my bodies so I was over flowing with energy. When I finish the spicy lemon-limeade cleanse not only did I crave healthier food, but I also was satisfied with smaller portions. When I crossed the ten day finish line I felt great because my body had been restored to a better state of health. I was delighted that after accomplishing the first ten days I established a new way of eating.

The spicy lemon-limeade cleanse influence our bodies to crave healthy foods. It regenerated our taste buds so we will not want to take another bite of unhealthy food loaded with salt, full of fat, chemically treated, or processed food. Breaking unhealthy food addictions can be very difficult that's why beginning your weight loss program with a quick and easy ten day detox cleanse with spicy lemon-limeade is a great way to get started.

How I felt after my spicy lemon-limeade cleanse is hard to put into words and it really has to be experienced to truly understand. When you get a taste of how good it feels to be truly healthy a mental awake you simply will not want to put unhealthy things in to your body again. The food we eat today are not like God intended them to be. Now they are filled with chemicals, hormones, drugs, and other impurity that gradual collect in our body over time and slowly poison us from the inside out. The spicy lemon-limeade cleanse can help flush away the years of waste that has been accumulating in our body.

I did not experience any hunger on my ten day cleanse since I was getting an adequate amount of calories daily, enough to fuel my body for the day. The objective isn't to starve ourselves skinny, the objective is to flush the toxins out and get healthy. 1 tablespoon of grape B maple syrup has 55 calories. There are also 4 calories in each tablespoon of lemon juice, 8 calories in each drink. If you use 2 tablespoons of the maple syrup in each drinks and you are drinking 8 glasses a day that provides a daily calorie intake of 944 calories or if you are drinking 12 glasses a day that provides a daily calorie intake of 1,416.

Benefits of Spicy Lemon-limeade

The spicy lemon-limeade is inexpensive to do and it only has four ingredients for the lemonade-limeade and is easy to prepare. Grade B maple syrup, organic lemons and/or limes, cayenne pepper, and filtered water. You will also need an herbal laxative tea and sea salt.

Grade B Maple Syrup - Grade B maple syrup is the most minimally processed of the maple syrups, making it more nutrient-dense. It contains trace minerals, which aids enzyme and antioxidant, zinc, supports immune systems, calcium aids metabolism, strengthens teeth and bones, helps regulate muscle, and heart contractions. It also contains magnesium, iron, copper, chlorine, sodium, nicotinic, pantothenic acid as well as vitamins A, B1, B2, B6, C. Grade B maple syrup also boosts your energy levels.

Cayenne Pepper - Cayenne pepper is a very good source of vitamin A, vitamin C, vitamin B6, manganese, and vitamin K. Cayenne is a known circulatory stimulant; it stimulate our body's circulation and reduces acidity. It also increases our lymphatic and digestive rhythms. It helps decrease appetite and slows the growth of fat cells. Studies on cayenne pepper indicates it also helps the body's thermogenesis which is the production of heat and it aids in the increase of lipid oxidation. Lipid oxidation is when fat is burned for energy. By heating the body the natural process of detoxification is streamlined. Cayenne is great metabolic-booster, aiding the body in burning excess amounts of fats. Cayenne is a well-known digestive aid. It stimulates the digestive tract, increasing the flow of enzyme production and gastric juices. This aids the body's ability to metabolize food and toxins, assisting the body in burning excess amounts of fats as well as normalize glucose levels. In addition cayenne pepper helps produce saliva, which is important for excellent digestion and stimulates intestinal motion, and aiding in elimination.

Lemon Juice - Lemon juice has Vitamin C in which helps to neutralize free radicals linked to aging and most types of disease. Lemon also have small amounts of thiamin, riboflavin, vitamin B-6, pantothenic acid, calcium, iron, phosphorus, potassium, copper and manganese. Lemons are alkaline-forming on body fluids helping to restore balance to the body's ph. The lemon is a stimulant to the liver and dissolves uric acid and other poisons, as well as liquefies the bile. Lemons help produce bowel movements thus eliminating waste. They also have powerful antibacterial properties and they destroys intestinal worms.

Lime Juice - Lime juice is rich in vitamin C and flavonoids a wonderful source of antioxidants which reduce the number of free radicals as well as detoxifies the body. Lime juice is a source vitamins A, E K, vitamin B1, B2, B3, B5 B9, and B6. The B6 vitamins help you metabolize the nutrients in foods. Limes are also a good source of calcium, magnesium, iron, copper, phosphorus, selenium, zinc, and potassium. The high potassium content of limes is very effective in removal of the toxic substances which get deposited in kidneys and the urinary bladder. There disinfectant properties relieves constipation. Lime juice is also excellent weight reducer. In addition limes are good for digestion they have a mouthwatering scent that supports digestion.

Spicy Lemon-limeade Cleanse Ingredients

The main ingredients can be found at most grocery stores. Keep in mind that the goal of the spicy lemon-limeade is to remove toxic substances from our body so stay away from ingredients that have been sprayed with pesticides. That is why it is extremely important that you use only organic ingredients and don't make any substitution from the ingredients listed below.

Organic lemons and/or limes
Organic cayenne pepper
Organic maple syrup grade B
Filtered water
There are a few really important things to remember when preparing the spicy lemon-limeade.

1. The lemon and/or lime juice must be fresh squeezed.
2. The maple syrup must be grade B.
3. Cayenne pepper is a necessary ingredient.

Terri Flynn

Chapter 6

Part One, Two & Three of the Cleanse

Part One of Cleansing the Holy Spirit's Temple

The first ten day consist of the spicy lemon-limeade cleanse.

Spicy Lemon-limeade Recipe

Make one glass at the time and always use freshly squeezed lemon and/or lime juice, then add the grade B maple syrup, cayenne pepper, and filtered water, mix then drink immediately. Keep in mind the longer your spicy lemon-limeade sits, the more enzymes are lost.

The lemon-limeade consists of:
2 tablespoons of organic fresh squeezed lemon and/or lime juice
2 tablespoons of organic grade B maple syrup
1/8 teaspoon cayenne pepper powder
8 ounces of filtered water

You should drink a minimum of 64 oz. 8- 8 oz. glasses of spicy lemon-limeade each day, but you can drink up to 12 glasses a day. Also drink as much water and decaffeinated herbal teas as you want.

Spicy Lemon-limeade Concentrate

I like to make a lemon-limeade concentrate for the entire days' worth of drinks. This way at the end of the day I

45

know how many glasses I consumed. Plus it is convenient if you are going to be out for the day. The concentrate consists of just two ingredients, the fresh squeezed lemon and/or lime juice and the grade B maple syrup. The maple syrup acts as a preservative for the enzymes in the lemons and limes. This lemon-limeade concentrate will keep the enzymes alive long enough to be consumed during the day.

Preparing Lemon-limeade Concentrate Recipe

Make 8 – 8 oz. servings
In a mason jar or a glass jar with a tight lid place
16 tablespoons of fresh squeezed lemon and/or lime juice
16 tablespoons of grade B maple syrup
When you are ready to have an individual serving of your spicy lemon-limeade add 1/8 teaspoon of cayenne pepper and 4 tablespoons of the concentrate to 8 oz. of water and enjoy.

Going out for the day

I pack a small cooler with ice when I am out for the day. I bring my mason jar with my lemon-limeade concentrate, cayenne pepper, 1/8 teaspoon, 1 tablespoon, a glass to mix the lemon-limeade concentrate in and a half a gallon of water.

Daily Bowel Movement

Bowel movements are essential to flush out the waste. Bowel movements is the process that cleanses your body of toxins. Since you are not consuming solid foods or fiber to create a bowel movement you may have to help that process.

Herbal Laxative Teas

Drink a cup of herbal laxative tea the night before you start your cleanse and every night that you are on the cleanse. Laxative herbal tea before bed will produce a morning bowel movement. One of the natural laxative found in many herbal laxative tea is Senna leaf. The leaf contains an herbal stimulant called sennosides that create a laxative effect on the body. Senna leaf has a sweet flavor somewhat similar to anise or fennel. Some teas that contain senna as a main ingredient are Laci Le Beau Super Dieter's Tea and Traditional Medicinal Smooth Move. The laxative tea will help flush out your system and will speed up the detoxing process by helping your body eliminate waste.

A.M. Salt Water Cleanse

In addition to the laxative tea you can also do a salt water cleanse in the morning as soon as you get up. This is optional but I find it very helpful to eliminate toxins. Purchase a good sea salt like Real Salt sea salt, Pink Himalayan crystal sea salt, or Gray Celtic sea salt. Do not use table salt and make sure the sea salt is unrefined and not iodized. You will want to give yourself at least two hour before you go out when you do the salt water cleanse it take that long to flush the salt water mixture out of your system. So I recommend that you stay at home near a bathroom when you drink it. I do the salt water cleanse every other day while I am doing this cleanse. However, you could do it every morning if you like.

Salt Water Cleanse Recipe

2 teaspoons of real sea salt
1 quart of filtered water
Use a glass jar or a BPA free plastic bottle
Mix a solution of sea salt and warm water. Shake well and drink the whole container of salt water immediately. The first time it might be hard going down, but I found that the second day was much easier.

Overview of part one of the program the ten day spicy lemon-limeade cleanse.

- The night before your lemon-limeade cleanse drink a cup of laxative tea.
- The first day of your cleanse in the morning before drinking a lemon-limeade drink, drink a quart of sea salt water remain near the bathroom. The sea salt cleanse is optional but highly recommended. You can do this every morning or every other day.
- Throughout the day drink 8-12 glasses of the spicy lemonade or limeade drink.
- In the evening drink some herbal laxative tea.

Part Two of Cleansing the Holy Spirit's Temple

The next nine days consist of a liquid fast with whole fruit and vegetable juice smoothies, whole vegetable pureed soups, fresh squeezed juices, herbal tea and of course plenty of water.

Whole Food Fruit and Vegetable Fast

Whole juices are excellent way to continue the detox and cleansing processes after finishing the spicy lemon-limeade cleanse. Whole juices are made in a high power blender, instead of a juicer. Incorporating whole juice as part of a balanced diet is a convenient way to add additional nutrition to your diet; than ordinary juice because it contains more of the pulp and protein our bodies require. You can think of whole food juice as a meal in a glass. A serving or two usually meets the daily recommended intake of fruits and vegetables.

The Importance of Fiber

If you have been on your weight loss journey for a while, you know that it is not all about removing things out of our diet. Sometimes eating healthier mean adding things to our diet, such as pulp. Whole juice fruits and vegetables are blended into a drinkable liquid without removing the pulp. This juice will have a think smooth texture.

Pulp is the dry fiber parts of fruit or vegetable which does not contain liquid, Fiber is important for a healthy digestive system and it will help keep your bowel movements regular. Most people do not consume enough fiber in their diet. Drinking whole fruit and vegetable juice is just one way to slip a little more fiber into your diet. Also you will burn calories drinking high fiber whole juice as you digest it. Plus pulp also fills you up longer so a glass of whole fruit and vegetable juice should keep you satisfied for three to four hours. In addition, the sugar from the fruit is absorbed slower because of the fiber which will help keep your blood sugar levels more even, avoiding the spikes and crashes from drinking fruit juice without all the fiber.

Storing Whole Food Juice

You can store whole juice longer without losing too much nutritional value because the fiber that the fruits and vegetables initially came with is still in the drink itself. To preserve a whole food juice put it in a glass container like a mason jar filled to the brim. This keeps the air out, so that the juice will not oxidize. Seal the jar and drink it within 24 hours. You might need to shake it if the water separates. Whole food juice do not take long to prepare so you can make your juice in the morning or even the night before you go to bed so you can take them with you for the day.

Good Quality High Speed Blender

To make whole fruit and vegetable juice and whole food pureed soups you will need a good quality high speed blender. There are many different high speed blenders on the market today. I have a Blendtec blender and I love it, it was money well spent. I used it more than any other appliance in my kitchen and it is easy to clean up. Keep in mind when you have a good quality blender you are going to be more motivated to use it. Therefore, you will be consuming more fresh and whole foods. In addition, using a good quality blender makes the food so much more enjoyable to consume as they have a smoother consistency. A powerful high speed blender allows you to grind up anything from raw carrots, apple, and nuts in to a liquid form.

Part Three of Cleansing the Holy Spirit's Temple

The next twenty one days you will be eating a Daniel fast. It is a very healthy way to eat. The Daniel fast is a wonderful way to start a life changing practice of eating healthy; by nourishing your body "the Holy Spirit's temple" with healthy fruits and vegetable. The Daniel fast often produces significant health benefits and many people with weight struggles encounter success as they submit themselves to the Lord and change their eating habits. Genesis 1:29 tells us, *"Then God said, "I now give to you all the plants on the earth that yield seeds and all the trees whose fruit produces its seeds within it. These will be your food."*

The Daniel Fast is a partial fast that is based on a vegetarian diet. Vegetarian are describes a person who does not consume meat, poultry, fish, or seafood. The Daniel fast is a diet healthy; one based on whole foods and water. On a Daniel fast, you may eat a wide variety of whole foods including fruits, vegetables, root vegetables, dried legumes, nuts, seeds, whole juice smoothies, 100 percent pure fruit or vegetable juice, herbal tea, and plenty of water. Keep in mind you are on a fast so limit yourself to only three meals a day and avoid over-eating and snacking.

Vegetable

They can be fresh, frozen, dried, or juiced. Include all kinds of vegetables in your diet such as, artichoke, arugula, asparagus, avocado, bamboo shoots, bean sprouts, beet, bell pepper, bok choy, broccoli, brussel sprouts, green and red cabbage, capers, carrot, yuca, cauliflower, celery, corn, cucumber, eggplant, garlic, endive, fennel, ginger, green beans, string beans, wax beans, beets, collard greens, kale, mustard greens, spinach, swiss chard, turnip greens, hearts of palm, horseradish, jicama, kale, leeks, lemongrass. lettuce, mushrooms, okra, olive, onion, scallions, peas, snow peas, sugar snap peas, all peppers chili, hot, mild, sweet, plantain, potato, pumpkin, radicchio, radish, squash of all kinds, sweet potato, tomato, water chestnut, watercress, yams, and zucchini.

Eating vegetables help improve your weight-loss progress. This is because many vegetables are high in fiber and low in calories, making them good choices for people who are trying to lose weight. Also people who get more fiber through their diet usually weigh less and have less body fat than people who don't eat enough fiber-rich foods. According to the Centers for Disease Control and Prevention. Vegetables tend to be low in energy density. Energy density is the amount of energy or calories in a particular weight of food and is generally presented as the number of calories in a gram. Foods with lower energy density provide fewer calories per gram than foods with a higher energy density. For the same amount of calories, a person can consume a larger portion of a food lower in energy density than a food higher in energy density. By eating foods that are low in energy density and calories helps you feel full even when you eat fewer calories, making it easier to lose weight.

Keep in mind that non-starchy vegetables are lower in energy density than starchy vegetables. There are two types of vegetables starchy and non-starchy. Both types are part of a proper diet. However, non-starchy varieties can be eaten in abundance. While starchy vegetables contain more sugar, calories, and carbohydrates therefore, portion size needs to be small and not eaten that often. Starchy vegetables include corn, peas, plantains, potatoes, squash, beans, beets, carrots, pumpkins, and yams.

Serving Size:

Vegetables are packed with nutrients that is why it is important to eat a variety of vegetables types at least four or more servings daily. Vegetables serving size: one cup raw vegetables, one-half cup cooked vegetables.

Fruits and Berries

Fruits and berries are a key part of a healthy diet especially if you are trying to lose weight; without adding any unnecessary fats. They provide the energy and nearly every nutrient that our body needs to reduce weight. Fruits provide nutrients necessary for good health and maintenance of our body. They benefit our body greatly as they provide a natural sources of vitamins and minerals, which are essential for the proper functioning of the body. Eating fruit is a great way to get a range of antioxidant, vitamins, minerals, folic acid and potassium. In addition, eating fruit helps keep our skin young, it provides vitamin C, which is necessary for building collagen. Fruit is a healthy carbohydrate food because it is alkaline forming and they are naturally low in sodium. They are rich in dietary fiber they contain soluble and insoluble fiber, which helps keep our colon free of the toxins and also help to improve the functioning of the digestive tract.

53

Fruit makes an excellent and satisfying snack. Eating a piece of fruit can satisfy a sweet craving without any detrimental effects. Fruit is filling because it's filled with fiber and water many fruits have up to 90% water. That makes them an awesome weight loss food. Eating an apple 30 minutes before a meal will fill you up and prevent you from overeating. Fruits are naturally low in fat, sodium, and calories. They are cholesterol free.

Fruit can be fresh, frozen, dried, or juiced. Include all kinds of fruit in your diet such as, apple, apricot. banana, blackberry, blueberry, cantaloupe, cherry, coconut, cranberry, date, elderberry, fig, raisin, grapefruit, guava, honeydew, kiwi fruit, lemon, lime, mango, cantaloupe, watermelon, nectarine, olive, orange, clementine, mandarin, tangerine, papaya, passion fruit, peach, pear, persimmon, plum, prune, pineapple, pomegranate, tomato, avocado, red raspberry, black raspberry, star fruit, grapes, and strawberry.

Serving Size:

Since fruits are packed with nutrients it is important to eat plenty of fruits three or more servings fruit a day. Fruits serving size: one medium piece of fruit, one-half cup cooked fruit, and four ounces of fresh squeezes juice.

Legumes/Beans

Legumes can be eaten on your weight-loss program they are packed with essential nutrients. Legumes fits into the protein food group, since they are rich in protein. They are also very high in fiber and complex carbohydrates. As well as B Vitamins, and complex carbohydrates. In addition beans help keep you feeling full longer. Which can help you lose weight when eaten in recommended portions. Keep in mind beans are not low in calories and can lead to weight gain when consumed in excess.

Include all kinds of dried legumes in your diet such as, black bean, black eye peas, navy bean, cannellini bean, chickpeas, chili bean, fava bean, great northern bean, kidney beans, lima bean, pinto bean, red bean, and white beans.

Serving Size:

Measure your servings since a proper portion of legumes is probably much smaller than you may realize. One-quarter cup of cooked beans from the legume group.

Organic Soybeans

Dried organic soybeans are rich in protein, and a good source of calcium, iron, phytoestrogens and it is complete with all the amino acids and it is also a good source of omega-3 fatty acids, copper, manganese, molybdenum, phosphorus, and potassium, B vitamin, riboflavin, folate, vitamin K, and fiber. In addition, the fat in organic tofu or soybean is mostly polyunsaturated and monounsaturated fats, organic soy is cholesterol and lactose free. As well as low in calories. When choosing soy you should always stick with the organic dried soybeans, dry roasted soybeans, fermented tofu, or edamame. Edamame is the fresh green form of soybean before they have been dried. Fresh edamame are deep green in color usually still in their pods and they can be found in the frozen food section. I grow edamame in my garden every summer. They are very delicious and easy to prepare.

Serving Size:

The serving size for organic soybeans, edamame, and tofu one-half cup. Dry roasted soybeans serving is one-third cup.

Nuts and Seeds

Nuts and seeds are also high in protein and an excellent source of healthy oils like omega 3. Nuts and seeds include vitamin E, B vitamins, as well as essential minerals like magnesium, potassium, copper, iron, zinc, selenium, some amino acids, as well as, unsaturated and monounsaturated healthy fats. Nuts and seeds are a healthy snack. However, because nuts and seeds are high in oils, and carbohydrates, you only need a small handful of them to get a serving from the protein group. Calories can add up quickly and pounds and come back on if you eat too many nuts and seeds.

Nuts and seeds include almond, walnut, Brazil nut, cashew, chestnuts, hazelnut, macadamia, pecan, peanuts, pine nut, pistachio and all natural nut butter. Chia seeds, flaxseed, hemp seeds, poppy seed, pumpkin seeds, sesame seed, safflower, and sunflower.

Serving Size:

A serving size of nuts is one-third cup. The serving size for seeds is one-eight cup.

Spices, Herbs, Oils, and Vinegars

You can also include healthy oils, spices, herbs, and vinegar when preparing your food.

Spices and Herbs

There are many benefits from cooking with herbs and spices. Adding herbs and spices to your food gives your meals extra flavor and you also get health benefits because herbs and spices contain antioxidants, minerals, vitamins. In addition some herbs and spices can help you maintain a healthy body weight by promoting weight loss. So be very generous when adding the following spices to your food. Cayenne pepper, cinnamon, black pepper, mustard, turmeric, ginger, cardamom, cumin, coriander, parsley, cloves, ginger, and peppermint. I encourage you to branch out from salt & pepper and try all the wonderful herbs and spices available to create delicious dishes.

Coconut Oil

Coconut oil has wonderful health benefits. It tastes good and it has powerful health benefits because ilt is especially rich in a fatty acid called lauric acid, which is known to improve cholesterol. The fats in coconut oil can also speed up your metabolism, increase your energy levels, reduce hunger, and increase feelings of fullness, it is also known to reduce abdominal fat. Since coconut oil can reduce appetite and increase fat burning, it makes sense that it can also help with weight loss. When it comes to high heat cooking, coconut oil is the best choice because it is not vulnerable to the oxidative damage that occurs with high-heat cooking using other fats. The high percentage of saturated fatty acids found in coconut oil makes it extremely stable when exposed to heat and is highly resistant to free radical formation when used for cooking at any temperature. No other oil comes close to being as safe and healthy for cooking as coconut oil. However, it is high in calories so use olive oil sparingly. This oil is semi-solid at room temperature and it can last for months and years without going rancid. Make sure to purchase organic virgin coconut oil.

Extra Virgin Olive Oil

Extra virgin olive oil it is the next best choice after coconut oil for cooking. Olive oil has high percentage of monounsaturated fatty acids which makes olive oil relatively stable when exposed to heat. Olive oil is rich vitamin E and Vitamin K, and is high in phenolic antioxidants, Omega 6, Omega 3. However, olive oil is high in calories so use olive oil sparingly.

Vinegars

Vinegar helps enhance the flavor of foods and they are very low in calories. Using vinegar in place of higher-calorie salad dressings or sauces significantly helps reduce your overall calorie intake, which is beneficial to achieving and maintaining a healthy body weight. Use more vinegar in cooking for salad dressings, marinades coleslaw, and soups. Vinegar can add extra flavor to many dishes. The best vinegar to use for cooking is more a question of taste, since their nutritional value is relatively similar. You can completely change your vinaigrette simply by alternating between balsamic vinegar, red wine vinegar, rice vinegar, white vinegar or apple cider vinegar. Choose vinegars without the added sugar and apple cider vinegar with the mother in it.

Things Not to Include in Part Three

While on part three of the Daniel fast you are leave out all animal products including beef, veal, pork, bacon, ham, chicken, duck, lamb, venison, mutton, seafood and fish, all dairy products, including cheese, cream, butter, eggs, as well as highly refined foods like sugar, and all processed foods. As well as sweeteners, sugar, raw sugar, honey, syrups, molasses, and cane juice. All refined and processed food artificial flavorings, food additives, chemicals, and foods that contain artificial preservatives. Deep fried foods like potato chips, french fries, corn chips, shortening, margarine, lard.

Some Daniel fast plans include grains however, we will be omitting them for the next twenty one days. Since one of the goals on these programs is to lose weight. Then we will slowing introducing them back in to our diets. That said omit all bread , baked goods, pastries, cookies, cakes, all grains, including but not limited to all wheat, rye, barley, brown rice, millet, quinoa, oats, barley, grits, all pasta, rice cakes, popcorn, corn and flour tortillas.

Sugar

Consider these facts next time your sweet tooth kicks in. Sugar-filled foods are among the most-craved items in many peoples diet. However, sugary foods fill us up with empty calories and too much sugar in our diet makes us gain weight and leads to disorders like diabetes, heart disease, inflammation, and some cancers. Also sugar can also make you feel tired, shaky, weak, faint, headachy, confused, and mentally dull. To loss and maintain a healthy weight you should limit or eliminate altogether refined sugar in your diet. Keep in mind when you are filling up on sweets we are probably not eating enough fruits and vegetables which contain the much-needed nutrients our bodies require to fight off disease. To sweeten food while cooking try stevia, apricot jam, grape B maple syrup, and honey in small amounts. So next time you feel a sugar craving coming on, reach for a piece fruit first.

Psalm 104:14 tells us, *"He causes the grass to grow for the cattle, and herb for the service of man: that he may bring forth food out of the earth."*

Ending the Fast

One of the most important phases of fasting is ending it appropriately. How you break a fast is extremely important for your physical and spiritual well-being. That is why it is so important to end a fast gradually. Since our digestive system has gone without unhealthy and large quantities of food for forty days you may encounter reactions like an upset stomach and weight gain if you suddenly eat a full meal or unhealthy foods after ending a fast. Our bodies need time to adapt as we bring back foods we have avoided. Keep in mind you should not eat a large amount of rich, fatty, or high calorie foods immediately after a fast. Instead begin slowly with smaller portions and little by little increase the quantity each day. If you end your fast slowly, the beneficial physical and spiritual effects will result in continued good health and you will keep the weight off.

Start with adding brown rice, black rice, wild rice, steel cut oats, quinoa, eggs, fish, and poultry. Keep in mind if you start eating the way you were before you lost the weight on the fast you will gain it back quickly. You have worked so hard to take the weight off so make a resolution to stay the course by carrying on the healthy eating habits you created on the fast.

You can do this by eliminate the red meats, processed foods, sugars, dessert, breads, caffeinated drinks and fried foods. By eliminate the unhealthy food after the fast you will experience continued good health and keep your desired weight. When you continually make one healthy decision after another you will be blessed with victory.

In Genesis *1:29,* God said, *"I am giving you all the grain bearing plants and all the fruit trees. These trees make fruit with seeds in it. This grain and fruit will be your food."*

Chapter 7

Water

Water and Digestion

Water is our body's principal chemical component and makes up about 50% to 75% of our body weight. Water plays a critical part in our nutrition and health and every system in our body depends on water. Since all of the tissues in the body need water to function properly it is essential to our survival. Regular water consumption has many benefits to our health and diet. Our digestive system depends on an adequate amount of water to help with the breakdown of foods. Water carries nutrients to our cells, it is also necessary for the absorption of food, for the removal of toxins, it boosts our metabolism, and encourages weight loss. Drinking water actually flushes out water weight. You should be drinking enough water so that you use the bathroom once every hour.

Drinking warm water or at least room temperature water before or after eating a meal will help break down foods making them easier for you to digest. Warm water increases our body's internal temperature which therefore, increases the metabolic rate and the increase in our metabolic rate helps burn more calories. Warm water helps break down the food in our stomach and keeps the digestive system on track; allowing our bodies to absorb the proper amount of energy and nutrition from the foods we consumed. Drinking a cup of warm water first thing in the morning is wonderful for weight loss. A cup of warm water in the morning on an empty stomach can help cleanse our bodies by flushing out toxins as well as improve bowel movements and reduces constipation by breaking down foods so they can pass through our intestines easily. Stimulating the bowels by drinking warm water will help return our body back to normal functioning. That is why it is better for our digestion to drink warm water than cold water.

Cold water does the complete opposite than warm water because it actually has a negative effect on our digestive system because it hinders our body's ability to properly digest food. Drinking cold or iced beverages with or after a meal delays our body's ability to properly digest food by slowing down our body's digestive actions. Any cold beverages basically harden the oil in foods and as a result create fatty deposit in the intestine. So instead of our food being properly digested food goes through our digestive system improperly digested. Therefore, our bodies are unable to get the nutrients and energy from it that it needs.

Furthermore, cold beverages rob the nutrition of the food we ate. When we drink cold beverages our bodies have to use energy in order to warm up that liquid inside our body. This robs our body of the energy it needs to properly process the food we have eaten. Instead of functioning to get all the nutrition of the food our digestive system is instead functioning on regulating the temperature of the cold beverage.

Instead of ice water or other iced beverages, you should consider room temperature drinks or even warmer liquids, such as hot water with lemon or hot tea.

Remember to try not to drink beverages straight out of the refrigerator. If a beverage must stay chilled in order to keep, make sure you pour a glass and then wait until it has warmed to room temperature before drinking. Also when you are in a restaurant, be sure you tell you server no ice.

Infused Water

If you don't like to drink water alone that you can add a little flavor and create a nutritious beverage by preparing infused water. Drinking fruit infused water may help you drink your daily requirement. In addition, they taste delicious. Infusing water with fresh fruits adds nutritional benefit. As the flavor enters the water, some of the nutrients also enter the water. Lemons, lime, oranges, grapefruit, pineapples and berries all are excellent sources of vitamin C. Nutrients provided by cucumber include vitamin C, vitamin A, iron, calcium, vitamin K and potassium. For stronger flavored water, prepare fruit infused a day ahead and keep it in the fridge overnight. Sip these tasty drink throughout the day as part of your water intake.

How Much Water You Need

Water consumption vary by individual size. The formula used to be eight 8 oz. glasses of water a day "one size fits all." However, that calculation has changed. The amount of water we need depends on our size and weight, and also on our activity level. In general, you should try to drink half your weight in ounces every day. To determine your daily water intake, take your body weight in pounds, divide it by 2 and drink that many ounces of water each day. For example, if you weight was 200 lbs. then you should drink 100 oz. of filtered water each day.

Keep in mind if you're living in a hot climate or exercising a lot, you would need to drink more water since you are expelling water when you sweat. You should add 8 ounces of water to your daily total for every 30 minutes that you work out. So if you work out for 45 minutes daily, you would add 12 ounces of water to your daily intake.

Health Benefits of Lemon Water

Fresh squeezed lemon juice has an anti-fungal, and antibacterial properties, and also has an immune boosting effect. Lemons contain valuable nutrients, including B-1, B-2, B-6, riboflavin, bioflavonoids, calcium, phosphorus and magnesium. By squeezing the lemon juice in to a cup of warm water first thing in the morning will assist your liver to break down fats and supports a healthy immune system. Lemons also contain pectin fiber, which assists in fighting hunger cravings. Lemons are also full of vitamin C which aids in calcium absorption and gives a clearer, smoother, and brighter looking skin. The vitamin C nourishes and rejuvenates the skin from the inside. Since toxins need a way to escape from our bodies often it's through our skin by regularly drinking lemon water will aid in quickly removing those toxins. In just a few weeks of drinking lemon water you will notice an improvement with your skin's tone and texture.

Lemons also helps in shifting our bodies from a state acidity in to an alkalizing state. Lemon juice helps to maintain a proper balanced alkaline pH balance within our tissues and organs. Keeping our system slightly alkaline is a helpful way to prevent illnesses and disease. When our bodies become acidic, the symptoms can include joint pain, stiffness, insomnia, and inflammation. The buildup of uric acid wastes in our body occurs from a diet high in animal protein, processed foods, sugar, and starches.

Starting the day with warm lemon water can help dissolve uric acid in the joints, the reduction of uric acid and will assist our body to become slightly alkaline which will improve these issues. The citric acid from a lemon is like a water softener for the body which helps cleanses our tissues and is excellent for dissolving uric acid and harmful mineral deposits that damage our organs, tissues, and joints by removing uric acid in our joints, which is one of the main causes of inflammation. Also by drinking lemon water regularly it will help to increase alkalinity and decrease unhealthy bacteria. Since bacteria and viruses flourish in an acidic environment in the body an overload of acidity in the body can set in motion many health issues.

Lemons are full of alkalizing minerals such as calcium, magnesium and potassium. By drinking warm lemon water daily helps boosts alkalinity and overtime will begin to reverse symptoms of acidity, therefore, also reduce inflammation, arthritis, stiffness in the joints. Lemon water can also flushes out calcium deposits, kidney stones, pancreatic stones, and gallstones.

Lemon juice have a detoxification effect they encourage in the elimination, digestion, acts as a natural diuretic and cleansing process of our bodies. Lemons with warm water helps to eliminate waste from the body. It helps improve digestion, reduce constipation, diarrhea, and bloating. Lemon cleansing purities interacts with our digestive tract, they cleanses our system and allows food to digest properly. The bitterness of the lemon increases bile which acts as a natural laxative and stimulates the gastrocolic reflex which causes a bowel movement. Lemon water is similar to the structure of hydrochloric acid, bile and other digestive juices. Lemon water normalizes hydrochloric acid production in the stomach and helps control the excess flow of bile in the liver and promotes healthy liver enzyme levels. If you are experiencing digestive issues you will see a difference if you start your day with warm lemon water and drink a cup after each meals. In addition, lemon water is also known to help lower blood pressure and improve the cardiovascular system overall.

Terri Flynn

Chapter 8

Detoxification

A Detox

Detoxifying is the process of releasing accumulated toxins that build up in our bodies systems. This process occurs within our bodies on a natural and regular basis; our bodies do much of the detox process through perspiration, bowel movements, and urination. However, as we age and our immune systems weaken from unhealthy diet, pesticides, and preservatives, we sometimes need to give our systems some help.

Excess weight is one of the first signs that we have a toxic body. Toxicity is sometimes a result of consuming foods that do not work for our body. Which will result in poor digestion and toxic overload.

Keep in mind that everyone responds to detoxification process differently, depending on the level of toxicity in the body. Some problems you may experience from the toxins you have in your body can include migraines, inflammation, weight gain, constipation, headaches, food allergies, muscle aches, hormonal imbalances, fatigue, acne, and eczema.

While fasting, our body are able to cleanse out all it systems because it is not utilizing all its energy towards the digestive system. Fasting encourage our bodies to release toxins from our colon, kidneys, bladder, liver, lungs, sinuses, and skin that have developed from an unhealthy diet. As our body shifts into releasing toxins from cells and tissues, we need to reinforcement the courses of elimination by drinking plenty of water so that these toxins can make their way out of our system through bowel movements and urination.

A cleanse is a great way to learn more about ourselves and to tune in to our bodies by paying attention to the warning sign it provides us. One person can feel sick after beginning a cleanse another person may feel energized and renewed. In addition, you can experience withdrawal symptoms at the beginning of the cleanse program. Withdrawal symptoms are a good sign they are revealing that your body is eliminating toxin. These symptoms general go away in 3 or 4 days of starting the cleanse program. They can include bad breath, flu-like feeling, fatigue, irritability, Itchy skin, nausea, body odor, and difficulties sleeping.

For many people, the body will not begin to lose weight or reduce inflammation until it has found balance through the cleansing process. Keep in mind how and when weight-loss occurs varies for each person, since everyone comes into the detox with a different level of toxicity. During the cleanse program, even if you don't see much weight-loss in the beginning, hang in there. You're doing the preliminary work and once the toxins are removed the weight will begin to come off.

A cleanse helps the body re-balance itself and helps repair the damage done by unhealthy eating habits. When we try to lose weight without doing a cleanse program the weight-loss usually comes back quickly and often more then we loss.

Constipation

Bowel movements are key to a detox process. Having daily bowel movements will help make sure that toxins aren't reabsorbed into your system. Think of it like cleaning your house; if you don't clean your house on a daily bases, garbage will pile up quickly. Often bowel movements will increase during a detox however, sometimes you many experience constipation. If you find yourself constipated you are probably not drinking enough water or eating enough fiber-rich foods. There are some natural things you can take to have bowel movements. Such as, magnesium citrate, it will help restore your magnesium levels which will encourage bowel movements. I also recommend whole psyllium husk and bentonite. You can take these every night and they will encourage gentle bowel movements and helps maintain regularity.

Keep in mind that bowel cleansing will remove harmful toxic bacteria out of our body. However, it can also remove all the healthy bacteria. For that reason we need to restore the healthy bacteria back to the body. One way to do this is to take a high quality probiotic.

Natural Laxatives

Psyllium husk is one of the best dietary fibers. It will add bulk to your stool and works as a mild intestinal lubricant, and assists in the colon cleansing process by transporting the waste through the intestinal tract. Keep in mind that when psyllium comes in contact with liquid, it swells and becomes a gelatinous mass. So psyllium husk must be consumed right away. Psyllium should be a staple ingredient for your colon cleansing process. Studies have shown that high soluble fibers such as psyllium husk help lower cholesterol, reducing the chances of heart disease. Research also shows that dietary psyllium may help to increase the excretion of fat in the stool. In addition, psyllium enhances the feeling of fullness and reduce hunger.

Bentonite Clay

Bentonite clay is a medicinal powdered clay which is derives from deposits of weathered volcanic ash. Bentonite has a high concentrate of minerals including silica, calcium, magnesium, sodium, iron, and potassium. A bentonite cleanse is one of the most effective natural intestinal detoxifying cleanses. As the clay absorbs water the clay's particles swell, forming a large porous mass. As this indigestible mass moves through the intestinal tract, it acts as a parasite cleanser; it is an effective way of purging the body of accumulated parasites. Bentonite clay is a unique clay due to its ability to produce an "electrical charge" when added to waste. This negatively charged is moderately alkaline which bonds to the positive charge in many toxins. The clay effectively draws out positively charged acidic toxin, chemical, heavy metal, free radicals and pesticides that reside in the intestinal tract. When it comes in contact with the toxin that have attached to the intestinal tissue's walls, the clay will absorb the toxin and release its minerals for the body to use. The clays alkalizing and astringent effect also gently removes encrusted deposits of old mucus, fecal material, and helps balance gut bacteria by pulling the bacteria off the walls of the intestines.

Flax Seed

There are many benefits of ground flax seed. Flax seed contains both soluble and insoluble fibers. Flax seed is an anti-inflammatory; the soluble fiber in flax seed is highly effective in lowering cholesterol one of the added benefits of a colon cleanses with flax. Flax seed also has a lubricating and healing effect on the entire digestive tract. In addition, flax seed is the best known dietary source of lignans it has at least 75 times more lignans than any other plant food. Studies also suggests that flax seed can lower blood pressure. People who have had a heart attack are reported to benefit from diets rich in alpha-linolenic acid, which is found in flax seed.

Homemade Colon Cleanse

An effective, inexpensive, and easy to prepare intestinal parasite colon cleanse can be made out of bentonite clay, psyllium husk, and ground flax seed. This homemade concoction offers a gentle, pure, and natural cleanse. The bentonite clay will absorb the toxins and parasites, while the psyllium husk will keep the mass moving through the intestinal tract and out of the body. While on the forty day cleanse right before bed, combine one tablespoon of bentonite clay, 1/2 tablespoon psyllium husks, 1/2 tablespoon ground flax seed in to eight ounces of room temperature water then stir and drink quickly. Keep in mind that you should not drink the clay within two hours of medications or supplements as it might reduce their effectiveness. Also do not use metal utensils as it alters the bentonite clay's electric charge which is essential, because the electric charge is what allows the bentonite clay to draw out the toxins.

Free Radicals

Free radicals are simple molecules with an electron missing. They are an unstable molecule, one whose naturally paired electrons have been split up. In an effort to become whole again they seek out other chemical structures in our bodies from where they can take an electron. Once they take an electron the chemical structure of the tissue from where they grabbed that electron is left damaged.

Free radicals are created by oxidation and oxidation is unavoidable. Breathing oxygen causes oxidation in our body and as a result creates free radicals. Free radicals in small and controlled quantities are normal and indeed are helpful in everyday metabolism and they take part in normal reactions in the body. The problems start when the production of these free radicals increase and then get out of control; in excess they will speed up our aging and lead to all sorts of harmful health problems.

Antioxidants

Antioxidants are the disease-fighting compounds in foods to help our bodies stay healthy by protecting the body from free-radical damage. We can take advantage of those antioxidants by eating a variety of foods that are high in antioxidants. The best way to ensure adequate intake of the antioxidant nutrients is through a balanced diet consisting of foods high in antioxidants such as fruits, vegetables, legumes, nuts and seeds. Eating healthy will help battle the damage done by free radicals and help to fend off the free radical process.

Knowing which foods have the most antioxidants is important. The list below are delicious foods filled with antioxidants.

Broccoli contain antioxidants in the form of Sulforaphane. In addition broccoli is also a good source pantothenic acid, vitamin B1, B6, vitamin E, manganese, phosphorus, choline, vitamin A, potassium, copper, omega-3 fatty acids, zinc, calcium, iron, niacin, and selenium.

Apricots contain antioxidants in the form of lycopene and also has a good amount of and vitamin C, vitamin A, and carotenes. They are also good source of minerals such as potassium, iron, zinc, calcium, and manganese.

Cranberries contain antioxidants in the form of phytonutrients. Cranberries are a very good source of vitamin C, manganese, as well vitamin E, vitamin K, copper, and pantothenic acid. Keep in mind that dried cranberries have a lot of added sugar and sugar can help form free radicals.

Raspberries contain antioxidants in the form of Ellagitannins, phenols and anthocyanins. Raspberries are an excellent source of vitamins A, vitamins C, vitamins E and vitamins K. They are one of the best berries to eat for their antioxidant value.

Strawberries contain antioxidants in the form of phytonutrients they also contains a full day's worth of vitamin C. As well as vitamin A, vitamin D, vitamin B6, calcium, iron, and manganese

Blueberries contain antioxidants in the form of anthocyanin. Blueberries are a good source of vitamin C, copper, vitamin K, and manganese.

Blackberries contain antioxidants in the form of ellagic acid. It is also a good source of vitamin E, folate, magnesium, potassium and copper, and a very good source of dietary fiber, vitamin C, vitamin K, iron, and manganese.

Cherries contain antioxidants in the form of phytonutrients. Cherries are also a good source of vitamin C, vitamin A, calcium, protein, potassium, and iron.

Watermelon contain antioxidants in the form of lycopene. Watermelon also contains thiamin, riboflavin, niacin, vitamin B-6, folate, pantothenic acid, magnesium, phosphorus, potassium, zinc, copper, manganese, selenium, choline, lycopene, and betaine.

Oranges contain antioxidants in the form of vitamin C. Vitamin C is an antioxidant known for boosting our immune system. Oranges are a good source of B vitamins including vitamin B1, pantothenic acid, and folate as well as vitamin A, calcium, copper, and potassium.

Grapefruit contain antioxidants in the form of Lycopene. Grapefruit is also a good source of Vitamin C pantothenic acid, copper, dietary fiber, potassium, biotin, and vitamin B1.

Peaches contain antioxidants in the form of phenols and selenium. Peaches is also a good source of vitamin C, vitamin E and K, niacin, folate, iron, choline, potassium, magnesium, phosphorus, manganese, zinc, and copper.

Prunes contain antioxidants in the form of Phenols. Prunes is also a good source of magnesium, calcium, vitamin c, and vitamin K.

Apples contain antioxidants in the form of Polyphenols. Apples is a good source of potassium, phosphorus, calcium, manganese, magnesium, iron and zinc, vitamin A, vitamin B1, vitamin B2, vitamin B6, vitamin C, vitamin E, vitamin K, folate, and niacin

Cantaloupe contain antioxidants in the form of Polyphenols. Cantaloupe is also a good source of potassium, vitamin B1, vitamin B3, vitamin B6, folate, vitamin K, and magnesium.

Lemons contain antioxidants in the form of vitamin C and bioflavonoids. Lemons are an excellent source of potassium, calcium, fiber, vitamin B6, iron, magnesium, riboflavin, and thiamin.

Limes contain antioxidants in the form of source of vitamin C, Limes are an excellent source of phytonutrients, flavonoids, iron, calcium, and other trace minerals.

Tomatoes contain antioxidants in the form of Lycopene.

Tomatoes are also an excellent source of vitamin C, biotin, molybdenum, vitamin K, copper, potassium, manganese, vitamin A, vitamin B6, folate, niacin, vitamin E, and phosphorus.

Artichokes contain antioxidants in the form silymarin. Artichokes are also an excellent source magnesium, chromium, manganese, potassium, phosphorus, iron, and calcium, vitamin B, niacin, and vitamin B6.

Spinach has plenty of the antioxidants vitamin C. Spinach is also an excellent source of vitamin K, vitamin A manganese, folate, magnesium, iron, copper, vitamin B2, vitamin B6, vitamin E, calcium, potassium, vitamin C, phosphorus, vitamin B1, zinc, protein, and choline.

Corn contain antioxidants in the form of Lutein. Corn is a good source of pantothenic acid, phosphorus, niacin, dietary fiber, manganese, and vitamin B6.

Kale contain antioxidants in the form of beta-Carotene, and Vitamin C. Kale is a very good source of vitamin B6, dietary fiber, calcium, potassium, vitamin E, vitamin B2, iron, magnesium, and vitamin B1.

Bell Peppers contain antioxidants in the form of carotenoids. Bell peppers are also an excellent source of vitamin A, vitamin C, vitamin B6, folate, vitamin E, vitamin B2, pantothenic acid, niacin, and potassium.

Asparagus contain antioxidants in the form of glutathione. Asparagus is an excellent source of vitamin K, folate, copper, selenium, vitamin B2, vitamin C, vitamin E, manganese, phosphorus, niacin, potassium, choline, vitamin A, zinc, iron, protein, vitamin B6, and pantothenic acid.

Brussels sprouts contain antioxidants in the form of Sulforaphane. Brussels sprouts are an excellent source of vitamin C, vitamin K, folate, manganese, vitamin B6, choline, copper, vitamin B1, potassium, phosphorus, and omega-3 fatty acids.

Carrots contain antioxidants in the form of beta-Carotene. Carrots are also very good source of biotin, vitamin K, molybdenum, potassium, vitamin B6, vitamin C, manganese, niacin, vitamin B1, panthothenic acid, phosphorus, folate, copper, vitamin E, and vitamin B2.

Watercress contain antioxidants in the form of Vitamin C, vitamin-K, beta-carotene, lutein and zea-xanthin. Watercress is also rich in riboflavin, niacin, vitamin B-6, thiamin and pantothenic acid, copper, calcium, potassium, magnesium, manganese, and phosphorus.

Lentils contain antioxidants in the form of anthocyanin. Lentils are also an excellent source of molybdenum and folate, copper, phosphorus, manganese, iron, vitamin B1, pantothenic acid, zinc, potassium, and vitamin B6.

Pecans contain antioxidants in the form of an anthocyanin. Pecans are also an excellent source and vitamin E, vitamin A, vitamin B, vitamin E, folic acid, calcium, magnesium, phosphorus, potassium, and zinc.

Oats contain antioxidants in the form of Avenanthramides. Oats are an excellent source of manganese, molybdenum, copper, biotin, vitamin B1, magnesium, chromium, and zinc.

Gluten Free Diets

More and more people are eating a gluten free diet. Many people have a gluten intolerance. A gluten allergy is the body's inability to digest or break down the gluten protein found in wheat and certain other grains. Gluten intolerance or gluten sensitivity can range from a mild sensitivity to gluten to full-blown celiac disease. Gluten allergy sufferers cannot digest gluten products and it is because of this that they are experience unpleasant symptoms such as bloating, inflammation, cramps, gas, diarrhea, headaches, and weight gain.

Gluten is not a protein itself but rather a protein composite, which means it is composed of several different proteins. The primary proteins giving gluten its utility in baking and its difficulty in health are glutenin and gliadin (in wheat), secalin (in rye) and hordein (in barley). These are elastic proteins; in the protein family known as prolamins. This unique protein composite is insoluble in water and comes from the endosperm within the seeds of grass-related grains. In Latin gluten meaning glue, a substance that provides an elasticity and glue-like capacity to hold its flour products together and provide them with a chewy texture.

Wheat is one of the main staples of a Western diet and is an enemy for those with a gluten allergy. Maintaining a gluten free diet consist of staying away from all foods that contain wheat, barley, bulgur, rye or produces made from them such as, breads, pasta, crackers, bagels, cereal, pastries, wheat starch, wheat bran, wheat germ, couscous, cracked wheat, durum, farina, graham flour, semolina, spelt, and many processed foods. Oats themselves don't contain gluten, however, they are processed in plants that produce gluten-containing grains and may be contaminated. It is important to check what is in the food being bought to avoid gluten toxicity. Keep in mind that the list of gluten-containing grains doesn't end at wheat. Gluten may even be found as ingredients in chicken broth, malt vinegar, soy sauce, some salad dressings, veggie burgers, seasonings, and spice mixes.

Gluten free labeled foods can be just as bad as foods containing gluten because they swap the gluten for other starches including tapioca, potato, rice, and corn. These starches send our blood sugar levels through the roof and can also contribute to more belly fat, heart disease, and arthritis. Consider avoiding gluten free labeled foods as much as possible especially while you are on a forty day cleanse.

Eliminating gluten from my diet helped me with my weight loss. I was amazed how this simple change of removing glutens from my diet cause my body to switch into fat burning mode without feeling like I was on a diet. The inflammation and bloating stopped, and my belly started to slim down. When you are trying to lose weight, gluten should be reduced to a minimum in your diet or removed completely. Glutens also spike our blood sugar levels, which signals our body to store fat.

It may seem hard to go gluten-free at first. But for many people the advantages far outweigh the inconvenience. The list of off-limit items may seem overwhelming in the beginning. Thankfully, there are plenty of replacements on the menu. Lots of foods are naturally gluten-free, such as, fruits and vegetables, beans, seeds, legumes, nuts, potatoes, eggs, organic tofu, all rice, amaranth, arrowroot, buckwheat, millet, quinoa, organic soy, and oats.

Terri Flynn

Chapter 9

Calorie & Calculations

Calories

Calories are simply a measure of energy. Just as, a pound is a measure of weight and a mile is a measure of distance. Our body needs calories to function as it should. The amount of calories needed per day changes from person to person. How many calories we need depend on our body size, age, height, weight, activity level, and gender.

Food and beverage are our sources of calories and physical activity impacts the rate we burn those calories. There are many factors that affect how much weight can be loss. However, weight loss will only occur when the calories we burn are more than the calories we consume. Therefore, learning to control how much we eat and exercising more will allow us to establish a calorie deficit; only then will we start losing weight.

There are approximately 3,500 calories in a pound. This means that if we consume 3,500 more calories than what we burn we will gain one pound. On the other hand if we burn 3,500 more calories than we consume we will lose one pound. The average adult female needs between 1,400 - 2,000 calories a day and for males the range is between to 2,000 - 2,500. If we eats this amount of calorie in a day we would maintain our weight.

The Basal Metabolic Rate

The Basal Metabolic Rate (BMR) is an estimate of how many calories we burn in a 24 hour period; if we were to do nothing but rest. (BMR) represents the minimum amount of energy needed to keep our body functioning. This figure gives us the number of calories our body needs on a daily basis in order to operate as it should.

The example below is a simple formula to figure out how many calories you need per day. First you must determine your activity level before you can figure your calorie needed in a day. From the choices below pick which statement best describes your current activity level. Determining whether you should multiply by 10, 11, or 12 depending on your activity level.

(10) Not active life style or sedentary people; who have an office job, or who rarely, or never exercise.

(11) Moderately active life style; people who do physical work, or those who exercise, or play a sport 3 to 5 times a week.

(12) Vigorously active life style people; who do extremely physical work, or those who exercise, or play a sport daily.

Multiply your desired weight, not your current weight by the number that best describes your activity level to determine how many calories you need a day.

Example:

If you're not active or have sedentary life style and your desired weight is 115 lbs. X 10 (not active life style) = 1,150 calories needed per day.

If you're moderately active and your desired weight is 115 lbs. X 11 (moderately active life style) = 1,265 calories needed per day.

If you have a vigorously active life style and your desired weight is 115 lbs. X 12 (vigorously active life style) = 1,380 calories needed per day.

Body Mass Index (BMI)

Body mass index also referred to as (BMI). BMI is used to characterize different weight groups in adults 20 years old or older. BMI is a number calculated from a person's weight and height. This calculation helps us figure out if we are at a healthy weight for our height. The more body fat a person has the higher the number will be. The suggested upper limit of body fat as a percentage of body mass is 24.9. A BMI of 25 or above is said to be overweight.

Body Weight Assessment
Underweight: BMI is less than 18.5
Normal weight: BMI is 18.5 to 24.9
Overweight: BMI is 25 to 29.9
Obese: BMI is 30 or more

BMI offers a consistent measurement of body fatness for most people and is a screening tool to decide if our weight might be putting us at risk for health problems such as heart disease, diabetes, high blood pressure, high cholesterol, or high blood glucose.

Body Max Index Calculations

BMI can be calculated by using pounds and inches with this equation. For example, a person who weighs 155 pounds and is 5 feet 2 inches tall has a BMI of 28.4.

$$BMI = \left(\frac{155 \text{ lbs.}}{(62 \text{ inches}) \times (62 \text{ inches})} \right) \times 703$$

You can calculate your body mass index by using feet, inches, and pounds. The mathematical formula for calculating BMI is easy to figure out. I have provide a step by step examples below.

1. Measure your height in inches using the tape measure. (Example 5' 2" = 62 inches)
2. Multiply the number of inches by the same number of inches. (Example 62 inches x 62 inches = 3,844)
3. Divide your weight in pounds by the second figure (Example 155 1bs. divide by 3,844= 0.004032)
4. Multiply that answer by 703. (0.004032 x 703= 28.34496 round up to 28.4) This number is your BMI
5. According to the BMI 28.4 falls in the overweight range.

Terri Flynn

Chapter 10

Helpful Tools

Below are some tips to help you to control your hunger:

Ways to Control Hunger

When you are feeling hungry, ask yourself are you really hungry or are you eating because you're feeling stressed, bored, alone, or frustrated.

Eat often: Try to eat every 4 hours, eat smaller meal and if you have to eat snack let them be healthy snacks or whole food smoothies in between. By eating more often, your body stays in a higher-metabolism digesting mode.

Wait: When you are feeling hungry, before you start munching on everything in sight wait a few minutes. Make your hunger wait for at least 15 minutes. If you wait a few minutes your hunger will probably diminish. During that time read the Bible, pray, or keep busy.

Stay hydrated: Staying hydrate will help you feel full. Drink at least half your body weight in water each day. Include lemon water, fruit infused waters, and herbal tea into you water intake. Keep in mind it is best to drink room temperature water, since cold water slows digestion.

Be prepared: Keep low-fat snacks like vegetables and fruit nearby. Then if you must eat have a small piece of fruit or some raw vegetables.

Cut back: Eat smaller portion of food or at least the proper serving size.

Slow Down: Eat slowly and chew your food completely, this will allow time for your brain to tell you when you've eaten enough.

Get up: Leave the table before you are stuffed; you will feel more aware and satisfied.

Be Mindful: Stop buying unhealthy foods you are likely to indulge on.

Stop eating: 3 hours before you go to bed and give yourself a fourteen hours fast window.

Body Measurement Tracking

Measuring our body part shows us that we are building muscle and losing fat. Losing inches is a better indicator then pounds. What should happen when we begin a weight loss program is we should lose fat and replace it with lean muscle mass. Since muscle weighs more than fat we could lose a lot of fat in inches and not lose much weight on the scale. Therefore, the scale could remain the same because we may have lost two pounds of fat and exchanged it with two pounds of muscle. When we recognize that our body parts are getting smaller and we are losing inches, we are moving in the right direction.

When taking your measurements you will need a flexible fabric tape measure. When taking measurements, you need to measure with the same tightness and same spot every time so you will get an accurate measurement. The measuring tape should be well-fitting. If skin is starting to protrude out from over and under the tape measure, you are measuring too tight, and if it's moving around freely, you don't have it tight enough. Make sure to do it the same way every week.

Measures
Neck – Measure the smallest part of your neck.
Chest – Measure under your armpits and shoulder blades.
Arm – Measure the largest part of your arms.
Waist – Measure the s at the belly button.
Hip – Measure the widest portion of your hips.
Glutes - Measure the largest part of your glutes.
Thigh – Measure the fullest part of your thigh.
Calves – Measure the largest part of your calf.

Exercising

Exercise supports weight loss results and overall well-being. Exercise could be the most difficult step to follow. However, if you want to keep off the weight permanently physical activity is key. Start slowly and steady then increase the amount of exercise. For example, today you will walk for ten minutes, repeat this for an entire week. For the next week, increase it to twenty minutes. The important thing is that you are moving and that your heart rate is up.

Take the slow and steady approach. It took you years to get out of shape; give yourself time to get back into shape. Try to get at least thirty minutes of brisk exercise preferably nonstop every day. Exercising daily will not only help you to lose weight and help you to maintain a healthy weight but it will also help you:

Strengthen your heart and lungs

Increase the level of HDL (good) cholesterol

Helps get rid of the LDL (bad) cholesterol

Lower an elevated blood pressure

Prevent adult-onset diabetes

Keep your bones strong

Strengthen and tone your muscles

Improve your productivity and energy levels

Reduce stress

Reduce feelings of depression

Exercise should become as much a habit as eating or sleeping. Not only does exercise help curb appetites, but it also helps speed up our metabolism. A faster metabolism means extra calories are burned even after we've stopped exercising. In addition, exercise will help increase muscle mass and decrease fat tissue. The more muscle tissue we have helps burn more calories per hour than fat tissue, so the more muscle we add to our body, the more calories we'll burn.

When - The best time to exercise is before a meal.

Frequency - Exercising daily helps it to become a habit.

Intensity - You should feel slightly short of breath.

Time - 30 to 60 minutes a session is a good workout.

Type of exercise - Whatever kind of movement that you enjoy that will give you an aerobic workout such as walking, jogging, cycling, swimming, or low-impact aerobics routines.

Burning Calories While Exercising

Physical activity leads to immediate calorie distribution during a workout, and it helps us to continue burning extra calories even when our fitness routine is over. Physical activity also causes the muscles of the body to do more work and enlarges our muscle tissue, as a result physical activity raises the amount of calories we burn while resting; this is because muscle is more metabolically active than body fat.

The key to good health and weight loss is to burn as many calories as possible. To lose weight we need to increase our activity level which will help to burn more calories.

Walking

The Surgeon General suggests accumulated and moderate intensity physical activity such as walking for thirty minutes or more of at least five days per week to improve health. Accumulated means you can do it in shorter sessions throughout the day for example, three ten-minute intervals throughout the day. Moderate intensity means you feel warm and slightly out of breath when you do it.

A good average walking speed is three miles per hour. However, it depends on your leg length and how quickly you can move your legs. Once we exceed four miles per hour, it is considered speed-walking. Keep in mind you may need to start at a slower pace if you're out of shape, but you will build up your speed quickly if you walk regularly. Treadmills produces the same benefits and is a great way to get your walking in if you cannot go outside.

Aerobic & Anaerobic Exercise

The word aerobic means with oxygen. Aerobic exercise refers to an intense physical workout that causes oxygen to be delivered to the muscles through the lungs and blood supply. Aerobic activities include speed walking, jogging, swimming, jump rope, roller-blading, rowing, dance, and tennis. Aerobic training is often called cardio exercise because it strengthens the cardiovascular heart and respiratory systems.

The word anaerobic means without oxygen. Anaerobic exercise refers to fitness routines such as lifting weights, that don't rely on oxygen for fuel. Anaerobic workouts typically involve short bursts of energy, which are powered by non-oxygen fuel sources stored in the muscles called adenosine triphosphate and glycogen.

The ideal calorie-burning training program involves a combination of both anaerobic and aerobic exercises. As a guide if you are doing a sixty minute workout divide your program into a forty minutes cardio and a twenty minutes weight-training, or you could do aerobics one day and weights the next.

Stretching

Stretching stimulate the flow in our lymphatic system and as a result cleanse our immune system. It also increases our range of motion, helps prevent injuries and, increases flexible.

Stretching tips:
Don't stretch too far
Don't bounce
Stretch slowly and hold it in a comfortable position
Exhale as you stretch and breathe slowly and naturally
Stretch after a workout when muscles are warm

Conclusion

Keep in mind that fasting should redirect our appetite from food to God. It help us to see that Jesus is more pleasing than eating. The pleasures of the stomach are decreased to enjoy the pleasures of the soul. Philippians 3:19 "*Their destination is destruction, their god is their appetite, their glory is in their shame, their minds are set on earthly things.*" When we allow our physical appetites to rule our life, and we can't imagine anything better than food, we are allowing food to become an idol. However, through fasting and prayer we begin to make Jesus the center of our life and we begin to see things differently. We begin to see food as a gifts from God. We begin to enjoy growing in fellowship with Jesus more than pleasing our appetite.

Never fast for the sake of fasting; fast for the sake of Jesus. Dieting and fasting both involve saying no to some foods, however, the goals are different. When we diet we seem to care more about the physical bodies than about the spiritual bodies. A diet limits food for physical reasons; but a fast limits food for spiritual reasons. Fasting is not just a self-improvement project. However, you will experience a healthier and leaner you at the end of these forty days. But that is a benefit not the end goal. Real fasting is turning attention away from ourselves and turning our attention to Jesus. The moment fasting loses its Jesus focus, fasting loses its value.

Fasting helps us get closer to Jesus; it is where our emptiness meets God's fullness. Every one of us is made in such a way that nothing can fully satisfy our hunger except for Jesus Himself. When we are fasting we should not just be limiting food but we should also feasting on the

Word of God. Fasting is all about seeking and finding fullness in Him. It is a way to practice what Matthew 4:4 tells us, "Jesus replied, "It's written, *People won't live only by bread, but by every word spoken by God."* While fasting, we should be skipping physical food to make room for spiritual food.

Fasting is also a way to seek a greater joy, to be hungrier for Jesus more than for food. Psalm 4:7 tell us *"You brought me more happiness than a rich harvest of grain and grapes."* Fasting is a physical expression of spiritual desire. When we fast, we are saying to Jesus we enjoy Your gift of food, but we enjoy the Giver even more. For the next forty days focus less on the gift and more on seeking the Giver.

As we eat the correct foods without excesses, our body will receive all the needed vitamins. Since God has already created all the needed vitamins and minerals in a perfectly balanced form, only these natural foods in their original form will bring us energy and sustain a healthy body. Therefore, we have no need for vitamin-enriched foods, unnaturally created for extra minerals. All refined and processed foods must be completely eliminated from our diet if we want to continue to be healthy.

One of the best things you can do during this fast is hide the scale, limit weighing yourself to once a week. Keep in mind how you feel is a wonderful gauge of success. So don't stress yourself out by stepping on the scale every day. The Lord wants us to experience both His provisions and His peace not to stress out over how much we have lost during the fast. Take the next forty days and start treating your body like God's temple, because it is God's temple.

Free Online Diet Support Sites:

Diet support sites to help you stay on track with your weight loss.

http://nutritiondata.self.com
http://www.calorieking.com
http://www.sparkpeople.com
http://www.fitclick.com
http://www.caloriecount.com
http://www.nutritionquest.com
https://www.supertracker.usda.gov
http://www.livestrong.com/myplate
http://www.health-alternatives.com
http://www.bmi-calculator.net
https://cronometer.com
https://www.myfitnesspal.com
http://www.fitday.com
http://www.loseit.com

Chapter 11

Recipes

Whole Juice Recipe

Use a high speed blender. Start by adding the liquid to your blender, followed by the soft fruit, add the greens or harder ingredients last. Blend on high for sixty seconds or until creamy. Consider adding one tablespoon of ground flax seeds or chia seeds. You could also add vanilla plant-based protein powder to many of these recipes.

Kale Pineapple Ginger
1/2 cup pineapple
1 large cucumbers
1 cup kale
1/2 lemon, squeezed
1/4 inch of ginger
1 cup filtered water

Coconut Chai
1 cup coconut milk
1 tbsp. vanilla extract
1 tsp ginger
1 tsp cinnamon
A pinch of allspice
2 tbsp. almond butter
1/4 cup shredded coconut

Blackberries pineapple
1 cup blackberries
1 cups of pineapple

1 cup coconut milk or almond milk

Peaches and Cream
1 cup peaches
1 cup coconut milk or almond milk
1 tsp freshly grated ginger

Pear Carrot
2 pears
2 carrots
2 stalks celery
2 nectarines, cubed
1 lemon, remove the rind
1/2 cups honeydew
1 orange remove rind
1 inch piece ginger
1 cup filtered water

Mango Watermelon
1 mango, peeled and pitted
1 cup watermelon
1/2 cup cantaloupe
1/2 cup honeydew
1 cup of filtered water

Pineapple Spinach
1 cup pineapple, cubed
1 cup fresh spinach
1/4 cup fresh parsley
1/2 teaspoon of fresh, grated ginger
1 cup of filtered water

Tropical Fruit
1/2 mango, peeled and pitted
1/2 cup papaya
1 small banana
1/2 cup pineapple
1 cup of filtered water

Orange Blackberry
1 cup blackberries
1 banana
1 small orange remove rind
2 cups fresh spinach
1 cup filtered water

Black and Blueberry
1 cup blackberries
1 cup blueberries
1 small apple
1 banana
2 cups spinach
8 ounces filtered water

Blackberry Melon
1 cup blackberries
1 cup watermelon
1 banana
2 cups spinach
1 cup filtered water

Mango Blackberry
1 cup blackberries
1 large mango, peeled and pitted

2 cups fresh spinach
1 cup filtered water

Red Blackberry

1/2 cup blackberries
1/2 cup raspberries
2 bananas
2 cups fresh spinach
1 celery stalk
1 cup filtered water

Apple Blackberry

1 cup blackberries
2 small apples
2 cups fresh spinach
1 small carrot
1 stalk celery
1 cup filtered water

Pineapple Avocado

1/4 avocado
1 cup pineapple
1/2 pear
3 cups fresh spinach
1/2 cup of filtered water

Kale Grapefruit

1 fresh squeezed grapefruit
1 cup kale
1 small apples
1/2 cup pineapple, cubed
1/2 cup of filtered water

Cabbage Grapefruit

1 fresh squeezed grapefruit
1 cup red cabbage
1 banana
1/2 cup of filtered water

Cucumber Grapefruit

1 fresh squeezed grapefruit
1 medium cucumber, peeled and sliced
1/2 cup fresh squeezed orange juice

Strawberry Grapefruit

1 grapefruit juiced
10 strawberries fresh or frozen
1 banana
2 cups baby spinach
1/2 cup of filtered water

Orange Mango Grapefruit

1 fresh squeezed grapefruit
1 orange
1 large mango, peeled and pitted
2 cups fresh spinach
1/2 cup of filtered water

Ginger Carrot Grapefruit

1 fresh squeezed grapefruit
2 medium carrots
1 teaspoon freshly grated ginger
1/2 cup of filtered water

Kiwi Apple Grapefruit

1 fresh squeezed grapefruit

1 apple
2 kiwifruit, peeled
1 banana
2 cups fresh baby spinach
1/2 cup of filtered water

Cantaloupe Fig

2 cups cantaloupe, cubed
3 fresh figs
3 cups fresh spinach
1 mango, peeled and pitted
1 cup filtered water, coconut water, or almond milk

Red Grape Fig

5 medium, fresh figs
1 cup red grapes
3 cups fresh spinach
2 bananas
1 cup filtered water, coconut water, or almond milk

Banana Fig

2 bananas
3 fresh figs
2 cups fresh spinach
1 cup filtered water, coconut water, or almond milk

Peach Fig

1 large organic peach chopped
3 fresh figs
2 cups fresh spinach
1 cup filtered water, coconut water, or almond milk

Apple Cranberry
1 cup of whole cranberries fresh or frozen
1 apple
2 cups fresh spinach
1 cup filtered water

Grape Cranberry
1 cup of whole cranberries fresh or frozen
1 cup red grapes
2 cups fresh spinach
8 1 cup filtered water

Banana Cranberry
1 cup of whole cranberries fresh or frozen
1 banana
2 cups fresh spinach
1 stalk celery
1 cup filtered water

Kale Cranberry
1 cup of whole cranberries fresh or frozen
1 cup frozen blueberries
1 banana
2 cups kale
1 cup filtered water

Strawberry Cranberry
1 cup of whole cranberries fresh or frozen
1 medium banana
1 orange, peeled
4 frozen strawberries
1 cup filtered water

Mango Blueberry

1 cup blueberries
1 mango pitted
2 cups baby spinach
1 carrot
1 cup filtered water

Banana Blueberry

1 cup blueberries
1 bananas
1 stalk celery
2 cups spinach
1 cup filtered water

Apple Blueberry

1 cup blueberries
1 apple
2 cups spinach
1/2 avocado
1 cup filtered water

Peach Blueberry

1 cup blueberries
1 peach
2 cups spinach
1/2 avocado
1 stalk celery
1 cup filtered water

Blueberry Apple

1 cup blueberries
1 large apple
2 cups spinach

10 medium strawberries
1 cup filtered water

Blueberry Pineapple

1 cup blueberries
1 cup pineapple
1 cups fresh spinach
1 banana
1 cup filtered water

Peach, Blueberry, Cucumber

1 cup frozen blueberries
1 medium banana
1 small peach, pitted
1 cucumber, with peel
2 cups baby kale
Juice from 1/2 lime
1 cup filtered water

Mango Coconut

1 mango, peeled and pitted
1/2 lime remove rind
1 banana
3 cups curly kale
1 cup coconut water

Orange Cream

1 large frozen banana
1/2 tsp. vanilla extract
1 fresh orange rind removed
1 cup coconut milk or almond milk

Pineapple Ginger Coconut

1 cup pineapple cubed
2 medium carrots
1/2 inch of fresh ginger root
1 cup coconut water

Infused Water Recipes

Spicy Cranberry Lemonade

1 cup of 100% cranberry juice
Fresh squeezed juice from 3 lemon
1/2 teaspoon cayenne pepper (optional)
Stevia to taste
Cut all the rinds from lemons in to thin slices
Place cranberry juice, juice from the lemon and the lemon
rinds in 1 gallon of filtered water, cayenne pepper

Cucumber lemon

1 cucumber cut in to thin slices
Fresh squeezed juice from 1 lemon
1 gallon Water
Cut all the rinds from lemons in to thin slices
Place cucumber slices, juice from the lemon and the lemon
rinds in 1 gallon of filtered water

Orange Grapefruit Lime

Fresh squeezed juice from 1/2 a grapefruit
Fresh squeezed juice from 1 Orange
Fresh squeezed juice from 1 lime
A few pieces of mint sprigs (optional)
1 gallon water
Cut all the rinds from fruit in to thin slices

Place the rinds and the citrus juice in 1 gallon of filtered water

Ginger Pineapple Mint

3 slices of Fresh Pineapple
1 tablespoon of thinly sliced ginger
1 gallon filtered water
A few pieces of mint sprigs to taste
Place pineapple slices, mint and ginger 1 gallon of water,

Ginger lemon Mint

Fresh squeezed juice from 2 lemon
 1 tablespoon of thinly sliced ginger
1 gallon filtered water
A few pieces of mint sprigs to taste
Cut all the rinds from lemons in to thin slices
Place the rinds, lemon juice, and mint and ginger 1 gallon of water

Hot Lemon Ginger

Squeeze 1/2 of a lemon in to a 4 ounces cup boiling filtered water with a few pieces of grated ginger, and stevia or a dash of honey.

Spicy Lemonade

Squeeze 1/2 of a lemon with a small pinch of ground cayenne pepper in to 10 ounces of filtered water, with a 1 tbsp. or grade B maple syrup

Soups

Lentil Lime Soup
6 cups broth vegetable
1 bay leaf
3 cups dried red lentils
3 tbsp. water
2 cups onions, chopped
3 garlic cloves, minced
3 tbsp. ground cumin
1 tbsp. turmeric
2 cups kale, finely chopped
1 cup fresh lime juice
Sea salt to taste

Rinse dry lentils in cold water until water runs clear. In a large pot, combine broth, bay leaf and lentils. Bring to boil. Reduce heat, cover and simmer for 30 minutes. In skillet over medium heat add onion, garlic, turmeric and ground cumin seed and sea salt with bit of olive oil or coconut oil and sauté until translucent. Mix sautéed onion spice mixture and chopped kale into the cooked lentils. Simmer for 15 minutes over a medium heat to blend flavors then add lime juice. Let cool slightly, pour mixture in to a high speed blender. Blend for 60 seconds or until soup has a smooth consistency. Serve warm.

Orange Ginger Carrot Soup
1 lb. bag of baby carrots
Juice from 2 oranges
1 inch piece of fresh ginger
2 cups vegetable broth

Place carrots in a pot with vegetable broth bring to boil, then simmer until tender. Let cool slightly. Pour carrots and broth in to high speed blender add ginger and orange juice. Puree until soup has a smooth consistency Serve warm.

Cauliflower Soup
1 tablespoon coconut oil
1 clove garlic, crushed
1/4 teaspoon ground nutmeg
1/4 teaspoon freshly ground black pepper
1 1/2 teaspoons sea salt
6 cups water
1 head cauliflower, chopped
1/3 cup chopped sweep onion

In a large pot over medium heat, melt coconut oil add garlic, nutmeg, pepper and salt and pepper cook for 30 seconds, Pour in the water add cauliflower. Bring to a boil, then reduce heat, cover and simmer 20 minutes, until cauliflower is tender. Pour cauliflower and broth in to high speed blender. Puree until soup has a smooth consistency Serve warm.

15 Bean Soup
1 - 1 lbs. package of 15 bean, dried beans
4 cups vegetable broth
1 tablespoon olive oil
1 large onion, chopped
1 garlic clove, chopped
2 celery stalks thinly sliced
2 carrots, thinly sliced
1 can diced tomatoes, undrained
8 tablespoons lemon juice

3 dashes Tabasco sauce

1 tablespoon oregano

2 teaspoons chili powder

2 teaspoons ground thyme

1 teaspoon cayenne pepper

½ tablespoon ground black pepper

½ tablespoon salt

Soak beans overnight, or at least 8 hours. Drain and rinse. In a 2 quart pot cook beans in 2 quarts of water until slightly tender by simmering on the stove for about 1 1/2 hours. Shortly before the beans are done, sauté onion and garlic in oil until slightly brown. When beans are done, drain half the cooking water. Add all remaining ingredients and simmer, uncovered, for 40-60 minutes, stirring occasionally. Adjust seasoning to taste.

Vegetable Broth

2 red onions, roughly chopped

2 stalks celery, roughly chopped

2 tsp caraway seeds

2 tsp sea salt

Freshly ground pepper

1 cup sliced shitake caps

4 large cloves garlic, chopped

1 cabbage, roughly chopped

2 tbsp. paprika

2 tbsp. fresh oregano, chopped

8 sprigs parsley, chopped stems and leaves

1/2 cup parsley, chopped

2 quarts water

Place all ingredient in a 3 quarts pot. Simmer for 30 minutes, remove vegetables.

Terri Flynn

About the Author

Terri Flynn was born and raised in Kingston, New York. At age 12 a seed was planted in her heart that would slowly grow and mature to a passionate love for Christ. In 1999, she surrendered her life to Jesus and began to seek after God through fasting, prayer, and meditating on His promises. It was through these times of prayer and study that Terri discovered that God's promises apply to the spiritual, emotional, physical, and financial areas of her life.

A desire for the Word of God was rooted in Terri's life when she attended Spirit Vision Bible College; at which time she made a commitment to say yes to whatever God asked. She wholeheartedly believes in the Word of God and has a passion for praying and proclaiming His promises. She has faith that God has made promises to us in His Word and as believers we should trust His promises. Terri discovered the power to live victoriously by applying God's Word to her life and wants to support others to do the same. She published her first book God Delights in the Prayers of His Children, in 2013.

Terri is active in her local church, Free Chapel, and she considers it a privilege to serve as a volunteer. She believes that the blessings and talents she has been given should be used to bless others. She has served in children's, youth, marriage, women's, and prayer ministries, as well as other outreach ministries. She attended Spirit Vision Bible College, School of Discipleship, and Joy School of Ministry. She married Sean in 2007; they reside in Georgia with their blended family.

Proclaiming Faith in Christ as Savior and Lord

God's grace He has already done everything to provide your salvation. Salvation is a gift from God. Ephesians 2:8 tells us, *"For it is by grace you have been saved, through faith—and this is not from yourselves, it is the gift of God."* Your part is simply to believe and receive Jesus as your Lord and Savior. This is the most important decision you'll ever make. The prayer of salvation begins with faith in Jesus. When you're ready to become a Christian you'll have your first genuine conversation with God.

God's Word promises, in Romans 10:9-10, *"If you declare with your mouth, Jesus is Lord, and believe in your heart that God raised him from the dead, you will be saved. For it is with your heart that you believe and are justified, and it is with your mouth that you profess your faith and are saved."*

You must believe that Jesus is God's one and only son. Believe that there are three persons in the Godhead the Father, the Son, and the Holy Spirit. Believe Jesus was crucified for your sins, was buried, rose from the dead, and ascended in to heaven. Believe that you receive salvation through the confession of and repentance from your sins. Believe that salvation is found in Jesus alone and there is no other name by which we can be saved. Ask Jesus to be your Lord and Savior.

If you believe then pray this prayer below out loud in faith and accept God's free gift.

Prayer of Salvation

Heavenly Father, I know that my sins have separated me from You. I am truly sorry. I am ready to walk away from my past sinful life and toward You. Please forgive me and help me avoid sinning again. I believe that Jesus is Your one and only son, that He died for my sins, and that You raised Him from the dead. By faith in Your Word, I invite Jesus to become the Lord of my life from this day forward. Please send Your Holy Spirit to help me do Your will for the rest of my life. In Jesus' name I pray. Amen.

If you prayed this prayer and your repentance is sincere and your faith in Christ is genuine you are now a follower of Jesus, a child of God. God's Word promises that you are a new creation and your name is now written in the book of life.

Welcome to the family. I encourage you to find a church where you can be water baptized and grow in the knowledge of God through His Word, the Bible.

Send prayer request to: <u>PrayerRequests@TerriFlynn.org</u>

My Testimony

This is my testimony of how God ordained my steps as a young child and brought two little girls together to save a man's life. I am certain that God ordains every step we take. We all have a journey with a purpose and destiny that God has planned for us. My journey began when my family moved to a new neighborhood in Kingston, New York where I met my best friend Rose. Our paths crossed when God placed me in a home across the field from hers. I was 4 years old and she was 5. As we grew, we were inseparable sisters at heart. We had no idea what God had planned for us. Proverbs 20:24, "Man's steps are ordained by the Lord, how then can man understand His way?"

As I look back, I can see God's hand working in my life. God is always working things together for good, but not just for my good. Sometimes we are part of His working things together for someone else's good, but we don't know it yet. When I was around 8 or 9 years old God started whispering in to my spirt that I would one day give Rose a kidney. I was not sure why I was having this thought which just came out of nowhere. The thought that I would give Rose a kidney would come and go throughout the years. I would ponder on it for a while but I kept it to myself I never told anyone about it. I was afraid people would think that I was weird since Rose didn't need a kidney. I know now that God was preparing me for a journey later on in my life. Romans 8:28, *"And we know that in all things God works for the good of those who love him, who have been called according to His purpose."*

Many years had passed and a thousand miles separated us but our friendship remained strong, and the thought of giving up a kidney faded until June 2012. Then the Holy Spirit started speaking to me again about giving Rose a kidney. I could not get it out of my mind for the entire month of June. I started praying and asking God for guidance and wisdom. Why was I having these thoughts? What did they mean? Was Rose sick and unware of it? I needed God's direction. This thought was too strong to be nothing. One thing I've found out in life is that when I am following God's will and obeying His voice He will give me confirmation.

Then one Friday evening the first confirmation came. Rose called to give me the news that her husband Frank was in renal failure and needed a kidney. I was blown away, I was speechless. I quickly hung up with her and prayed asking God if He really wanted me to donate my kidney. I don't believe there are coincidences. Coincidences are really God's hand in our life. It is God speaking to us and giving us direction and confirmation. Proverbs 16:33, "*We toss the coin, but it is the Lord who controls its decision.*"

The next day my husband Sean and I are in the car with our daughters and out of the blue our girls started talking about donating a kidney. I quietly laugh inside and said "Lord, You have got to be kidding." So my family and I had a lengthy discussion about kidney donation. I asked Sean if he would consider donating a kidney and he replied "yes I would." Up to this point I had still not told my family or anyone about Frank or what I though God was telling me to do. I continued to pray asking God for guidance and wisdom. I did not want to say it out loud if God was not telling me to do it. Then I did some research and I watched a YouTube video to see what the surgery entailed. Then Sunday night I told Sean what I believed God was telling me to do. Sean immediately agreed that I should donate my kidney to Frank. So we were in agreement. That was my second confirmation.

Rose and Frank were together for 25 years before they got married in 2011. The Bible tells us that marriage bonds us together as one. Mark 10: 8 says, *"The two will become one. So they are no longer two, but one."* For that reason I would essentially be giving Rose a kidney, when I gave my kidney to Frank. This is because Frank and Rose are one flesh since they are married.

I called Rose to tell her what God had been preparing me to do and we both knew it was a miracle orchestrated by God. So I started undergoing various medical tests to determine if I was a match, and I was a match. That was my third confirmation. Next we needed to see if I was healthy enough to donate the organ responsible for filtering the body's blood; after many test the doctors conclude I was in good health. However, I was a little overweight to donate an organ without potentially endangering my own health. So I would need to lose at least 19 pounds, before they would consider me as a candidate. They will only transplant individuals within the normal weight BMI. Recognizing I could make a meaningful change in Frank's personal health was really a great motivator to get the weight off. I knew it was time for me to get serious. I turned to God and asked for His help since losing weigh over the past eight years has been a struggle for me. Then I came up with the weight loss program Ten – Nine – Twenty One; that helped me loss the weight without starving myself. I lost 27 pounds in 40 days, enough for me to be eligible to donate. I had no doubt that God's hand was arranging my steps for many years; preparing me for such a time as this.

It was happening, I was donating a kidney to Frank. The transplant surgery took place July 6th, 2015 and it was successful. Frank and I are both recovering well; the doctors are very pleased. God just amazes me how He is in every little detail. I was told before the surgery to expect a lot of pain. Because the spleen, stomach, and intestine lie near the kidney, they needed to be moved in order to remove the kidney and this causes a lot of pain after the surgery as they settle back into place. The surgery is done by hand-assisted laparoscopy using a two smaller incision in the abdomen and a vertical incision near the belly button through which a hand is inserted to hold and then remove the kidney. After the surgery I found out that my left kidney, the one I donated, had extra-long arteries. God knew before I was born that I would one day need extra-long arteries on my left kidney. Because my arties where extra-long the incision was made just below my bra line instead of near the belly bottom as a result none of the other organs needed to be moved out of the way. Most people need to take pain medicine at home for 3-4 weeks following the surgery because of the pain. However, the only pain I experienced was a soreness in my abdomen; it felt like I did too many crunches. So I was done taking the pain medicine by the time I was released from the hospital 4 days later. Psalm 139:13 tells us, "You are the one who created my innermost parts; You knit me together."

I just stand in awe of Jesus, He is my healer. I am so grateful God gave me the opportunity to give the gift of life. I don't consider myself a hero for what I did and I don't want any of the credit. I want people to look at Jesus. It's the strength that He's given me that enabled me to do this. I want all the glory to be directed at Him not me.

Enjoy this additional book from author Terri Flynn

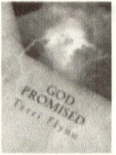

God Delights in the Prayers of His Children
Praying God's Word Back to Him through Scripture-Based Prayer

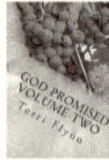

Twenty One Ten - Nine - Twenty One
More of Jesus, Less of Me Forty Day Challenge

God Promised
Proclaiming the Word Over

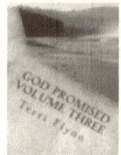

Volume One - Joy, Love, Faith, Peace, & Kindness

Volume Two - Worry, Anger, Fear, Anxiety, & Depression

Volume Three -   Prayer, Fasting, Giving, Strength, & Finances

Available for purchase online and as e-book
(God Delights in the Prayer of His Children) www.createspace.com/5176418
(Ten – Nine – Twenty One) www.createspace.com/5838774
(God Promised Volume 1) www.createspace.com/4926657
(God Promised Volume 2) www.createspace.com/5194452
(God Promised Volume 3) www.createspace.com/5213557

Visit me at:
terriflynnauthor.weebly.com
https://www.facebook.com/PrayerRequestsTerriFlynn.org

Terri Flynn